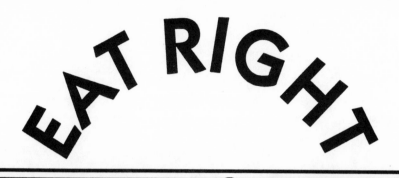

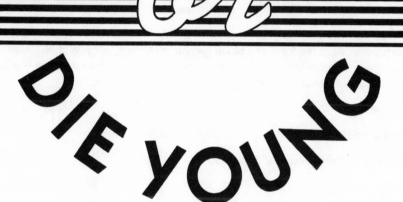

When Will YOUR Biological Clock Stop?

Dr. Cass Igram

with Judy K. Gray, M.S.

Instant Improvement, Inc.

Published by Instant Improvement, Inc., 210 East 86th Street, New York, New York 10028, with the permission of Literary Visions, Inc.

Fourth Edition

ISBN 0-941683-19-2

Printed in the United States of America

TABLE OF CONTENTS

PART I - PRINCIPLES

INTRODUCTION

What does it mean to die young? The human body is designed to live! How long? Well over 80, and up to 120 years. Yet many Americans are dying young. Diseases such as heart disease, cancer, and diabetes take their toll in premature deaths. Have you ever heard of or known a young, aspiring executive who, though apparently the picture of health, died suddenly and unexpectedly of heart disease? In all likelihood you have. Most all of us have at least one relative or friend who is afflicted with a life-threatening disease.

Regardless of all the hype about AIDS, cancer, and other killers, heart and circulatory diseases remain the number one cause of death in America today. This is despite the use of the most advanced methods of life-saving intervention known in the world. So why is there still such a problem? Surely, it is diet related.

Wherever the typical American diet exists, there too exists a high incidence of heart disease, diabetes, and cancer.

Poor diet and nutritional habits impair the function of the human body. Poor nutrition alters immune function, impairs circulation, and disturbs hormonal balance, resulting in disorders ranging from heart disease and arthritis to cancer. Faulty dietary habits predispose the body to all varieties of degenerative diseases, which I call *diseases of civilization.*

The worse the diet, the more likely it is that heart disease, stroke, heart attack, hardening of the arteries, high blood pressure, cancer or arthritis will develop. The longer an individual is on a poor diet, the more rapidly will such diseases occur.

A nutritionally depleted diet affects the gene pool as well. If your ancestors had a poor diet — a diet rich in refined sugars, white flour, processed foods, and refined fats — your genes will be affected. Then you will be even more vulnerable than they were to the development of the diseases of civilization.

The question is, why have a heart attack or stroke, or develop heart disease or cancer if you can avoid it? Isn't it better to prevent these things from happening? If you already have an illness, why not do something to attempt to cure it?

Modern medicine has led us to believe that there is no cure for the majority of diseases. Heart disease is a case in point. Most doctors claim the only thing that can be done is to "treat the symptoms." Or, they state that "eventually the patient will succumb to a heart attack or stroke, and

3

that the only known and effective treatment is by-pass surgery or medications." Regarding nutrition they claim, "Diet and nutritional supplements play a minor role, if any role at all."

I know these things are being said to my patients. If you have heart disease, the same has probably been said to you.

The medical profession takes the same stance for a variety of other disorders. Those afflicted with arthritis, cancer, skin diseases, colitis, peptic ulcer, and mental diseases are fed the same party line: "No cure exists except medications or surgery. Diet and nutrition play no significant role."

This fatalistic approach helps no one and may be harmful to many. It is a fact that these and many other conditions can be successfully treated through nutrition and dietary alterations. What may be even more important is that their development can be prevented by making specific dietary changes and by taking certain nutritional supplements.

Medical doctors do occasionally apply preventive measures. In the case of heart disease, some physicians give credence to exercise. Others insist upon avoiding naturally-occurring food substances, such as cholesterol, as a means of dietary treatment. Few, however, offer any hope for a cure.

At most, all these measures are just so many band-aids. The real causes behind disease and its development are not being addressed.

Those few, however, who do offer a cure are usually the surgeons. My definition of cure is certainly different from theirs. I believe in assisting the body's natural healing mechanisms thereby enhancing the instinctive curative powers found within every living cell and organ. By this definition, cures can be effected by feeding the body what it needs so it can heal itself. In contrast, surgeons claim that by removing the "diseased organ" they are effecting a cure. Thus, an individual with an inflammed or stone-filled gallbladder is "cured" once the gallbladder is surgically removed. No mention is made to the patient that there are non-surgical methods for curing gallstones or gallbladder disease. Nor is any mention made of the significant side-effects and illnesses which can occur months after the gallbladder is removed. The gallbladder was put there for a reason! Removing it *does* compromise certain bodily functions.

The cardiovascular surgeon and the cardiologist are particularly prone to proclaim curative powers. They actually make the claim to cure heart disease! The surgeon "cures" the angina and arterial blockage with his by-pass surgery, and the cardiologist performs the special "curative" procedure known as angioplasty. Here, cardiologists thread a tiny plastic tube (catheter) into the heart's arteries in an attempt to remove blockages.

There is no need for me to exert my personal opinion about the supposed curative power of these procedures. The statistics speak for themselves. Patients who refuse to undergo these procedures live, on the average, longer than those who do!

Internists also claim to cure. Drugs are given to patients who have high blood pressure in an attempt to artificially lower blood pressure. Ironically, artificially lowering the blood pressure can actually cause strokes. And this is the very thing these doctors are trying to prevent!

A government study showed that patients with moderately high blood pressure who were on blood pressure drugs died at a more rapid rate than those with high blood pressure who took no drugs. Blood pressure drugs exert their effect, in part, by a bizarre mechanism of action. They remove from the body the minerals necessary to maintain normal blood pressure!*

MEDICINE-FREE DOCTORING

Can a doctor practice medicine in the United States without using drugs? The answer is yes. Over a five year period, I treated people with a wide range of conditions. My prescription pad was used more often to write notes to airlines or for school excuses than for drug prescriptions. And I never used a hospital once during that period. There are many countries where drugs play a secondary role to natural, safer remedies such as herbs, diet, vitamins, minerals, etc. The same could be accomplished here. Unfortunately, much of the medical education is being influenced by the drug industry. However, some effort is being made to introduce nutrition into the medical curriculum. To be sure, the process is slow. If both the public and professionals work together, a dent can be made and medicine-free doctoring will become a mainstay.

Physicians need to be trained in the use of nutritional therapy. If this is done, eventually each person plagued with a serious illness will have the option to choose — to try safe, non-toxic therapies, or to go the route of modern medical care.

A life free of need for medications is a critical element in your attempt to live a longer and happier life. Death from over-medication can and does occur. The ill-advised use of potentially toxic medications, or dangerous surgical procedures is a major cause of premature death.

No doubt, medications and surgery are often useful and may even be life-saving during certain emergency situations. My argument is not against drugs or surgery per se, but against the claim that they cure. This is not true at all. It is the natural substances found within our food,

---

* Most blood pressure medications promote the urinary excretion of potassium, magnesium, sodium, and to a degree, B-vitamins such as riboflavin and vitamin B-6.

in our water, and on this earth that truly have curative powers. It may well be that for every malady, there also exists its cure or treatment. If you are having difficulty with this concept, understand that 85% of all medications currently being developed or used were originally derived from herbs. Many of these drugs are nothing more than man's attempt to synthesize (meaning "create" in a laboratory) what Nature has already created within the herb. Needless to say, the chemist cannot produce exact replicas of these natural healing agents. Vitamin E provides a good illustration of this. Researchers have found that natural vitamin E is far more potent and effective than its synthetic counterpart.

An excellent example of medical oversight concerns the treatment of the heart attack patient. Only recently was it discovered that the majority of hospitalized heart attack patients are deficient in magnesium. Most of our body's magnesium is found within the cells so the usual blood tests are not accurate. This is why magnesium deficiency in heart attack patients was not discovered earlier. Studies have shown that magnesium injections alone reduced the death rate by more than 90%! Is this common knowledge in our medical centers? NO!

Just think. This is but one of many naturally occurring substances. Imagine how healthy cardiac patients could become if all their deficiencies were corrected. Each health condition has its own specific nutritional deficits, as you will be shown later on in this book.

It has now been proven that high blood pressure is due, in part, to a potassium and magnesium deficiency. Does it make sense to take a drug which depletes the body of these minerals? Of course not. It makes better sense to restore the body's reservoirs of these critical nutrients.

Arthritis is often the result of a combination of weakened intestinal walls and intestinal toxicity. Does it make sense to treat arthritis with drugs which further damage the intestinal walls and increase the toxicity?*

Arterial blockage, when it occurs, reaches every artery system within the body. The body contains approximately 60,000 miles of blood vessels. Does it make sense, then, to clean out only the coronary arteries? Not at all. The sensible approach is to clean out all the arteries in the body.

Address the cause of whatever your condition is and you will feel better. Eat right and you will likely improve. Treat only the symptoms, and you may well die young.

* Arthritis medications, including Indocin, Clinoril, and aspirin, are known to cause intestinal bleeding. In fact, according to published reports in medical journals, arthritis medications are the #1 cause of emergency stomach or intestinal bleeding.

CHAPTER ONE
What Is Eating Right?

I t is just as easy to eat right as it is to eat wrong. I say this because most people feel that eating nutritiously requires more discipline than they could muster. They are afraid that eating right is synonymous with boredom and self-denial. Eating right does not imply these things at all. It means consuming only those foods or drinks which will help the body function better. It means avoiding all foods and drinks which are harmful to the body. This is a simpler and more meaningful way of looking at it. In fact, you are denying yourself *more* by eating what is harmful to you than by eating what is good for you. For example, would you purposely feed your cat or dog French fries, knowing full well that it could hurt it? If you wouldn't do this to your pet, then you most certainly shouldn't do it to yourself. Yet many people do.

Eating right, in essence, means not hurting yourself with YOUR OWN TWO HANDS! You are the one who chooses what you put in your mouth. Only you operate the controls. This book will help guide you to make the right choices.

WHICH CHOICE IS RIGHT FOR YOU?

What is nutritionally right for you may not be the same as what is needed by friends or relatives. Each person is genetically different, and the body's needs for certain nutrients may differ dramatically from one person to the next. For example, some people need 50 times as much vitamin B-6 as is usually required just to function properly.

Even so, there are some general rules of thumb which apply to virtually everyone. Throughout this book, I have outlined these rules. Without a doubt, there will be exceptions to the rules, but for the most part, 90% of all people will benefit by following my simple dietary principles.

KNOWLEDGE IS THE KEY

The key is to know which dietary habits can hurt you and understand why substances found in your diet are harmful.

Warning: Once you gain such knowledge, it becomes your responsibility to act upon it. Ignorance is not bliss, nor is premature death from a heart attack, stroke, or cancer.

YOU CAN EAT RIGHT — CHANGING OLD HABITS

Now you know the secret: knowledge. Use this book to your advantage and learn what is good and bad for you. Once you understand why certain things are harmful, it will be much easier to change old eating habits. You will find these habits easier to eliminate than you could have ever believed.

YOU CAN MAKE THE COMMITMENT

Commit yourself right away to changing any self-destructive habits you have. To do so, just follow these simple principles:

1. You are not responsible for ignorance, but as soon as you know right from wrong, you become responsible.

2. Do not hurt yourself with your own two hands.

3. Eating right is just as easy as eating wrong.

4. Since eating wrong is harmful, you are denying yourself more by eating wrong than by eating right.

Practice these principles. The rest of this book will give you the knowledge you need to follow them. This knowledge, together with a sense of responsibility for your personal health, will enable you to incorporate these principles into your lifestyle.

CHAPTER TWO
How To Eat Right

Eating right means eating naturally. It means that all foods and drinks consumed should be as close to their natural state as possible.

You might think you eat "right" now. But you probably don't. In all likelihood your subconscious mind has been polluted by the myth of the all-American balanced diet. We have been told over the last 40 years that the standard American diet of breads, grains, packaged foods, milk products, meats, vegetables, and fruits is entirely balanced in the nutritional elements we need. No account has been made for the method by which these foods are grown or processed — just as long as they reach your dinner table as a grain, starch, sugar, vegetable, fruit, or meat portion, that food will serve as an adequate part of the balanced diet. These foods have been divided into categories known as the four basic food groups. The fact that the foodstuff looks, smells, or even tastes different than it does naturally doesn't seem to matter. For example, instant potatoes most certainly taste differently than freshly mashed.

There are a number of loopholes in this philosophy. It is truly nothing more than a philosophy, since there is no scientific basis for the balanced diet structured upon the four basic food groupings. In addition, *no scientific studies have been done to support it!* First, almost no one knows what the four basic food groups are or what food elements they contain. For those who are unfamiliar, these food groups were created by food processors and their dietitians in the 1940s. Their idea was that if you ate at least one food from each group at every meal, your diet would be "balanced" in all the nutrients you need. However, even if you did know how to follow these principles, it is unlikely that you would be getting the nutrients you need.

Test yourself. Try to list the four categories on a piece of paper. If you can do so, list underneath each category the foods contained within it. I have yet to meet anyone, except an occasional registered dietitian, who knows this. Second, no attempt has been made to account for the variability in nutrient content as related to soil and growing conditions. Third, the damaging effect on nutrient content caused by food processing has not been addressed. Fourth, a more recent phenomenon, the fast food industry is currently playing the most predominant role in upsetting the principles of this philosophy. While a Big Mac or hot dog with an order of fries qualifies as containing three of the four basic food groups, any positive or nutritious benefits of such a meal are far outweighed by the damaging ones.

You are not eating right if you regularly eat fast foods, deep fried foods, processed, packaged, or canned foods, white flour, pasta, pastries, or sweets. You are not drinking right if you regularly consume pop, sugar-sweetened fruit drinks, cow's milk, or alcoholic beverages.

ARE YOU NUTRITIONALLY DEFICIENT?

If you follow the standard American diet, your eating habits are creating severe nutritional deficiencies. Here are the consequences of the all-American diet:

- 79% chance you are deficient in folic acid
- 70% chance you are deficient in niacin
- 62% chance you are deficient in vitamin B-6
- 70% chance you are deficient in thiamine
- 40% chance you are deficient in riboflavin
- 33% chance you are deficient in vitamin B-12
- 100% chance you are deficient in chromium
- 100% chance you are deficient in manganese
- 65% chance you are deficient in calcium
- 76% chance you are deficient in magnesium
- 75% chance you are deficient in selenium
- 100% chance you are deficient in essential fatty acids

The myth of the balanced diet is finally exposed! How can this be true? Very easily. Food processing destroys nutrients. This has been proven. For example, heating and boiling food can destroy over 90% of the folic acid content. You can bet there is little or no folic acid left in canned vegetables or in French fries which are cooked at searing temperatures of up to 400 degrees. The same is true for most other nutrients.

WHAT ABOUT FORTIFICATION?

There is little value to food fortification. The only commonly eaten processed foods which are fortified are the grains. In addition, the fortification process itself is incomplete. Only a few of the nutrients destroyed by processing are replaced. For example, in the process of converting whole grain to white flour some 24 nutrients are destroyed. Of these, the only ones replaced are thiamine, niacin, riboflavin, and iron. Few are aware that much of the vitamin E, vitamin C, vitamin A, and the minerals copper, chromium, manganese, magnesium and zinc are destroyed or left behind in the bran and germ during the milling process. The same is true for other refined foods such as white rice, corn meal, rye flour, oats, or barley. Let's look at this in terms of percentages.

VITAMIN LOSSES IN THE REFINING OF
WHOLE WHEAT INTO FLOUR

B-1 (Thiamine) ..... 77% is lost   Pantothenic acid .... 50% is lost
B-2 (Riboflavin) .... 80% is lost   Folic acid .... 67% is lost
B-3 (Niacin) .... 81% is lost   Vitamin E .... 86% is lost
B-6 (Pyridoxine) .... 71% is lost

MINERAL LOSSES IN THE REFINING
OF WHOLE WHEAT INTO FLOUR

Chromium .... 87% is lost   Zinc .... 82% is lost
Manganese .... 90% is lost   Iron .... 81% is lost
Copper .... 66% is lost   Magnesium .... 83% is lost

From the above you can see that most of us have significant nutritional deficiencies. This is because refined wheat and wheat products form a major part of the typical American diet. Add to this the consumption of vitamin or mineral destroyers, and the deficiencies can become profound or even life-threatening.

VITAMIN-MINERAL DESTROYERS

Are you using vitamin-mineral destroyers? This test will tell.

ANSWER YES OR NO TO THE FOLLOWING. DO YOU USE?

1. alcohol	2. antibiotics
3. aspirin	4. birth control pills
5. caffeine	6. cigarettes
7. coffee	8. cortisone
9. drugs	10. laxatives
11. mineral oil	12. water pills (diuretics)
13. white flour	14. white sugar

Count up the number of times you answered yes. If you only use one or two of these and your use is occasional, then you are probably destroying a small amount of nutrients. But if you regularly use any of these agents, you are at risk for severe nutritional depletion. If you use most or all of them, you are really in trouble! In this case, you are at risk for developing a variety of diseases due to extreme nutritional deficiencies.

MEDICATIONS ROB SPECIFIC NUTRIENTS

If you take prescription or non-prescription drugs, it is important that you carefully read this section. The medication you take may be causing deficiencies of specific nutrients. This is due to the fact that the mechanism of action of each drug is different. Most drugs are highly specific according to where they act in the cellular chemistry and in how they inactivate or destroy certain nutrients. The end result is that medications can be the primary cause of nutritional deficiencies. Here are some of the ways medications do this:

1. by increasing urinary excretion of nutrients

2. by blocking where the nutrient attaches within the cell

3. by blocking absorption of the nutrient

4. by binding to the nutrient and, therefore, inactivating it

5. by causing the nutrient to be used up more rapidly

6. by actually destroying the nutrient

7. by increasing the loss of nutrients in the stool

TABLE FOR COMMON MEDICATION-INDUCED DEFICIENCIES

This chart provides a comprehensive list of the major nutrients and the drugs which negatively affect them. There are hundreds of other drugs which cause these nutrients to be deficient — only the more commonly used ones have been included. The more drugs that are taken, the greater the odds that nutrients are deficient. Those taking a preponderance of medications, such as nursing home occupants, heart attack patients, etc. are likely to be deficient in most, if not all, of these nutrients.

DEFICIENT NUTRIENT	MEDICATION
Vitamin A	antacids, aspirin, cholestyramine, Coumadin
Vitamin B-12	antibiotics, aspirin, birth control pills (BCPs), cortisone, Mycolog, Stelazine
Vitamin C	antihistamines, aspirin, BCPs, cortisone, Coumadin, Indocin, tetracyclines
Calcium	aspirin, Phenobarbital, tetracyclines
Vitamin D	barbituates (Phenobarbital, Seconal, etc.), cholestyramine, cortisone, Dilantin
Vitamin E	BCPs, cholestyramine
Folic acid	antacids, antibiotics, aspirin, BCPs, Dilantin, Macrodantin, Methotrexate, sulfa drugs (especially Septra and Bactrim), Tagamet
Iron	aspirin, Clinoril, Coumadin, Indocin, tetracyclines
Vitamin K	antibiotics (all types), barbituates, cortisone, Coumadin, Dilantin, Pro-Banthine, tetracyclines
Magnesium	diuretics (including Lasix, Diuril, and Thiazides), laxatives, tetracyclines
Potassium	aspirin, cortisone, diuretics
Pyridoxine (vitamin B-6)	BCPs, cortisone, Dilantin, Penicillamine, penicillin
Riboflavin (vitamin B-2)	antacids, antibiotics, BCPs, diuretics, sulfa drugs

Thiamine (vitamin B-1) . . . . antibiotics, aspirin, BCPs, drugs
                                          containing caffeine, Indocin

Zinc . . . . BCPs, cortisone, drugs containing
                                          caffeine, diuretics

As is illustrated in the above chart, many non-prescription drugs cause nutritional deficiencies. Aspirin is one of the worst offenders. Another example is mineral oil. It binds to the fat-soluble vitamins such as vitamins A, D, E, and K, causing their loss into the stool. Other harsh laxatives, if taken regularly, cause deficiencies of vitamins and/or minerals. Regular use of antihistamines results in vitamin C and B-vitamin deficiencies.

Most people who take drugs are already nutritionally compromised. It is obvious that drugs make an already bad situation even worse. With drug therapy, little is cured and a lot is lost. On the other hand, nutritional therapy along with proper diet is safe and the gains are usually immense.

DR. IGRAM'S SEVEN WORRY-FREE PRINCIPLES FOR EATING RIGHT

I think you can see how important it is to begin eating right as soon as possible. Through improved diet, the body's nutritional reservoirs can be built up — the result being improved health. There are hundreds of opinions as to just what is the most nutritious diet. You are probably wondering how you can sort through all these opinions and the confusion they generate so you can learn to eat right. Following these principles will help simplify your task:

1. Do not worry about what you have eaten in the past. Just **eat right** from now on.

2. Do not worry about eating out. Just eat around the unhealthy foods.

3. Cooking foods is OK as long as you do not heat them excessively. Just try not to overcook your meats or vegetables.

4. Do not be concerned about eating all raw foods. Just eat some raw fruits or vegetables every day.

5. Do not worry about eating too much meat. Just avoid eating smoked, processed and preserved meats (i.e. bacon and other meats containing added nitrates).

6. Do not worry about eating an occasional canned or packaged food. Just try to eat as much food in its original, natural state as possible (for example, fresh beets versus canned).

7. Do not worry about food-combining or food groups. Just eat a variety of healthy foods.

CHAPTER 3
What Does It Mean
To Die Young?

Dying young is something most of us fear. There is nothing more scary than the thought of dying in a fiery car accident or in a plane crash. Though we don't usually think about it, most of us would like to live a normal lifespan. The degree of anxiety, with regard to premature death, depends on the type of illness a person has and also the severity of that illness. For those afflicted with heart disease, there is often a constant apprehension about dropping dead from a heart attack. Those who have cancer are concerned that the condition will eventually lead to their demise. Yet, dying young doesn't just mean living a shortened life span. It means living in a way that disrupts optimal productivity, both mentally and physically. By this definition, most individuals in nursing homes have "died young."

I equate living like a semi-vegetable with no purpose or function as a form of death. A person placed in a nursing home at, say age 60, despite living there until 80 years old, is dead, spiritually, emotionally, and to a large degree, physically at age 60. The cold, hard facts? Maybe. Yet, you know as well as I that this is what happens.

Is there any difference between death and a state of living death? I believe not. Examine your heart and see how you really feel about it. Chances are you dread the thought of living in a nursing home, no matter what the circumstances or provisions.

Modern medicine and emergency life-saving care are setting the stage for the elderly to live in this manner. I have seen individuals hooked up to tubes on respirators, living like mutes for up to 2 years or more, only to die as soon as the breathing tubes are removed. This is not what most of us have in mind for quality living. Dying young is just that: the loss of all quality of life. Thus, a morbidly ill cancer victim is dying young; a patient permanently disabled by a stroke or neurological disease, such as multiple sclerosis, has died young; an individual whose brain is fried by Alzheimer's or Parkinson's disease, has been lost before his time.

Premature death due to disease is dying young. The death of all children who have contracted cancer and were killed by either the cancer or the therapy, the death of all youths from alcohol and drug-related accidents, the loss of all women who, in the prime of their lives developed breast, ovarian or cervical cancer, the loss of vital, valuable men from heart attacks — all are examples of premature death.

What makes this subject so important? After all, these people are dead and gone. Nothing can be done about it. While this is true, the fact remains that many of these deaths could have been prevented. Also it is important to we learn from these events so that terrible mishaps can be prevented in the future. Believe me, most of these horrible deaths could have been prevented. If you are grieving for one of these precious souls, you will appreciate what I have to say.

Modern medicine is directly responsible for a certain percentage of premature deaths. It is well known that many medications can be toxic, especially if they are given in improper dosages. Thousands of people die or are permanently disabled every year as a result of the side effects of prescription medications. Up to 40% of the admissions in major medical centers across the country, are due to the side effects of drugs. Thousands of others die as a consequence of unnecessary surgical procedures. The irony of it all is that many of these illnesses could have been treated with much safer and less toxic therapies. Most diseases, if caught early enough, are treatable by methods other than drugs, surgery, or other invasive methods.

For those afflicted with a condition for which no treatment has yet been discovered (such as the loss of limb or spinal paralysis), I extend to you my love and support. For anyone else who is ill, I extend only this: do your utmost to get back your health. Continue to search for a solution. If you do, you will unchain your inner spirit, and what an excellent feeling that will be. For it is likely that you will live life to its fullest and avoid the plague of dying young.

CAUSES OF PREMATURE DEATH

A list of the more common conditions which cause premature death and/or significantly reduce the quality of life includes:

1. Alcoholism
2. Alzheimer's disease
3. Cancer
4. Diabetes
5. Drug addiction
6. Heart Disease
7. Neuromuscular diseases (i.e. multiple sclerosis, ALS, and muscular dystrophy)
8. Parkinson's disease

9. Rheumatoid Arthritis   10. Stroke

Nearly all of these diseases are preventable. Our environment, lifestyle, and diet are involved in generating these horrifying illnesses. By removing the causative factors and taking the appropriate treatment, one can expect to avoid becoming a victim of any of these diseases. Some of these diseases are so powerful that once you get them, little or nothing can be done to stop the progression. But everything can be done to prevent them from happening. Let's look at how you can stop them from striking you. You will find many pearls of wisdom throughout the book on how you can avoid disease, disability, or premature death which can result therefrom.

CHAPTER 4
Is Your Body
Giving You Signals?

Now it is clear how poor diet leads to nutritional deficiencies within the body. Once these deficiencies become severe enough, your body may give off certain warnings or signals. The body is wonderfully constructed, and one of its miracles is to provide us with warnings of impending danger. Many outward signs of disease or deficiency, while occurring often, are frequently overlooked by both the patient and the doctor.

Take dandruff, for example. This is a complex symptom, signaling a number of nutritional deficiencies. Dandruff, in its more severe form, is known by the medical term, *seborrhea* or *seborrheic dermatitis*. This term is derived from the oil-secreting *sebaceous* glands located in great numbers on the scalp. To make an adequate supply of their protective oils, these glands are reliant on a generous supply of substances known as *essential fatty acids*. In addition, their proper function depends on adequate supplies of the B-vitamins, especially B-6, niacin, and biotin. Dandruff is a reliable indicator of vitamin B-6 deficiency.

In summary, dandruff or seborrhea is associated with deficiencies in the following nutrients:

1. essential fatty acids
   (linolenic and linoleic acid)
2. vitamin B-2 (riboflavin)
3. vitamin B-3 (niacin)
4. vitamin B-5 (pantothenic acid)
5. vitamin B-6 (pyridoxine)
6. biotin
7. folic acid
8. selenium
9. zinc

As the deficiencies become prolonged and more severe, the local and systemic immunity becomes diminished. Thus, the hair follicles and sebaceous glands become infected. This occurs particularly when there is a B-6, zinc, and essential fatty acid deficiency.

It has now been established that scalp disorders, notably seborrhea, psoriasis, and simple dandruff are all associated with the overgrowth of a fungus which normally inhabits the scalp. Other microbes such as the bacteria strep and staph may play a role. A diet high in sugar worsens these conditions. Those little flakes of dandruff are a warning that your nutritional state has gone awry.

The body may give off other warnings. You might notice changes in the texture and color of your hair or it may become excessively oily or dry. Dry or oily hair is a tell-tale sign of essential fatty acid deficiency. Your hair is a barometer of the nutritional state of your body. It is particularly sensitive to changes in fatty acid and protein nutrition. Changes in your hair can be noticed shortly after a period of intense emotional stress. In susceptible individuals, just eating a few servings of deep fried foods can lead to noticeable changes in the health of the hair and scalp.

Unmanageable hair which stiffens and stands out on its own is a classic sign of poor fatty acid nutrition. Hair loss is indicative of vitamin-mineral malnutrition along with poor digestion and absorbtion of fatty acids and proteins. Excessive hair loss may also be a signal of impaired blood flow to the scalp.

Although most people eat plenty of protein, that doesn't mean it is being digested and absorbed properly. If this is the case, the hair, being mostly protein, will reflect it by signals such as hair loss, split ends, slow growing hair, and brittle hair. The health of hair is also dependent on another group of nutrients: minerals. Most important in this regard are zinc, sulfur, and silicon.

The fingernails, though representing a small surface area, provide all sorts of indications about what is going on inside the body. Ridges on the nails often indicate hormonal disturbances. Thumb-nails that look like spoons are accurate indicators of iron deficiency and, therefore, anemia.

The skin can be revealing. Patches of dry, scaly skin, particularly on the face and cheeks indicates poor fatty acid, zinc, and B-6 nutrition. Easy bruising without trauma may signal a deficiency of vitamin K, bioflavinoids (found in fruits and vegetables, especially the rinds of citrus fruits) and vitamin C.

There are, of course, signs of a more serious nature which can occur. Pain in the chest, arm (particularly the left one), shoulder, or jaw may precede a heart attack. A hardened, fixed mass in the breasts may forewarn of breast cancer. Changes in bowel habits may be an early warning of bowel cancer. These *medical* signs require medical diagnosis and treatment. Is your body giving you signals that you are developing significant nutritional deficiencies? Take this test to find out.

CHECK THE APPROPRIATE RESPONSE	YES	NO
1. Do you have dandruff or seborrhea of the scalp?	☐	☐
2. Is your hair dry or brittle?	☐	☐
3. Do you have premature graying of the hair?	☐	☐
4. Is your hair losing its texture or shine?	☐	☐
5. Is your hair excessively oily?	☐	☐
6. Do you have alopecia or significant hair loss?	☐	☐
7. Does your skin crack open easily, especially during the winter?	☐	☐
8. Do you have acne?	☐	☐
9. Do you have dry patches of skin on your face and cheeks?	☐	☐
10. Is your skin dry and flaky?	☐	☐
11. Do your fingernails grow slowly?	☐	☐
12. Do your fingernails break or peel?	☐	☐
13. Do you have white spots on your fingernails?	☐	☐
14. Do your fingernails have ridges?	☐	☐
15. Do you have hangnails?	☐	☐
16. Are your hands and feet always cold?	☐	☐
17. Are your eyebrows falling out (especially the outer third)?	☐	☐
18. Are you developing growths on the skin such as moles, skin tags, raised brown spots, etc.?	☐	☐
19. Do you bruise easily?	☐	☐

20. Do your gums bleed easily or do they
    bleed when you brush?   □   □

21. Are you developing age or liver spots?   □   □

INTERPRETATION OF RESULTS

If you answer yes to any of these signals, you have nutritional deficiencies. Some of these are more serious than others. The following is a listing of what each means medically and nutritionally.

#1 As stated earlier, you may have an overgrowth of fungi and bacteria in the scalp secondary to both nutritional deficiency and a breakdown in immunity. Most of the B-vitamins are lacking, especially B-6, niacin, biotin, and folic acid. Deficient minerals include zinc and selenium (many dandruff shampoos contain selenium as the active ingredient). Essential fatty acid deficiency and protein maldigestion are likely.

#2 Major factors: protein maldigestion/deficiency and essential fatty acid deficiency. Vitamin A is also probably lacking. Brittle hair indicates mineral deficit, especially sulfur.

#3 Major factors: stress is a biggie. B-vitamin deficiencies are likely, especially vitamin B-5, PABA, and folic acid. A hormonal imbalance should be considered.

#4 Major factors: a lack of essential fatty acids seems to be the key. Deficiencies of B-6 and zinc are also associated.

#5 Major factors: both oily and dry hair are associated with a malabsorption and/or deficiency of essential fatty acids. Zinc, B-6, and folic acid are also lacking.

#6 Major factors: poor circulation to the scalp is a common causative factor. Alopecia (patchy hair loss) may be a sign of heavy metal poisoning. Alopecia is also associated with deficiencies of folic acid, zinc and inositol (a natural substance not technically listed as a vitamin or mineral). Hair loss and/or balding is a sign of severe deficiency of a wide range of nutrients, including protein, essential fatty acids, B-vitamins, silicon, and zinc.

#7 Major factors: a severe deficiency of essential fatty acids is almost certain. There may be a malabsorption or deficiency of essential amino acids. This symptom may also be a sign of adrenal dysfunction.

#8 Major factors: nutritional deficiency and acne go hand in hand. This is especially true if the acne is in teenagers. It is likely that the diet is poor, being high in fried foods, saturated fats, and refined flour and sugar. Food allergies also play an important role. Vitamins that are deficient include B-2, B-3, B-5, B-6, A, C, and E. Improving essential fatty acid nutrition will help clear the acne as will supplementing with minerals, especially zinc and potassium.

#9 Major factors: this is a sign of essential fatty acid, zinc and B-6 deficiency.

#10 Major factors: this is a classic indication of severe essential fatty acid, zinc, and B-6 deficiency. When fatty acid nutrition becomes this poor, other internal problems develop. Metabolically active organs become damaged, and they may actually degenerate or shrink in size. These highly active organs include the liver, thyroid, and adrenal glands. The heart and arteries are also affected. Without an adequate supply of these fatty acids, circulation becomes reduced. The cells lining the digestive tract are dependent upon a plentiful supply of essential fatty acids. These cells die and are renewed every 3-8 days. Without the nutrients they need, they will not form properly. When this happens, malabsorption of the nutrients from our food will result. If your skin is poor in quality and is dry and peeling, just think about how your insides look! The same degenerative process is likely going on within you as well.

#11 Major factors: this is indicative of protein, fatty acid, and mineral malnutrition. The minerals most commonly lacking are calcium, magnesium, sulfur, and zinc. Vitamin A also plays an important role.

#12 Major factors: calcium deficiency is definite, although essential fatty acids play an important role. Other needed minerals include zinc, magnesium, and iron. Brittle nails in women may signal iron deficiency anemia. A severe vitamin A deficiency is also likely.

#13 This indicates zinc deficiency. Malabsorption of zinc due to a lack of pancreatic enzymes is also probable. Vitamin A deficiency can also lead to zinc malabsorption, since a healthy intestinal absorptive surface is dependent upon an adequate supply of it.

#14 Ridges are an indication of severe nutrient malabsorption, especially protein and minerals (sulfur and calcium), although hormonal imbalances are also involved.

#15 Major factors: folic acid and vitamin A are the most important deficiencies indicated by this sign. Hang nails are usually cured when these two nutrients are taken in a sufficient dosage. In essence, hang nails are an indication that the body is not able to synthesize the cells which line the inside and outside of our body fast enough. These cells are known medically as *epithelial cells*. Vitamin A and folic acid help restore the rate of synthesis of these cells back to normal. Zinc may also be necessary to maximize the rate of cellular repair.

#16 Major factors: it is likely that the thyroid and adrenals are malfunctioning. This may also be a clue to vitamin E or essential fatty acid deficiency. Patients with yeast infections often have cold extremities. So do patients who are deficient in vitamin A and/or niacin (vitamin B-3).

#17 Hypothyroidism is almost definite if you have this. If prolonged or left untreated, this condition can result in a variety of problems including fatigue, weight problems (too heavy or too thin), elevated cholesterol, cardiac arrhythmia, chronic fungal infection (in the intestine, vagina, or on the skin), digestive disturbances, cold extremities, etc.

#18 The development of new growths on the skin is a sign to take seriously. While it may not mean you have cancer, such growths are a warning that serious problems such as cancer could occur. This is particularly true if you are developing new moles, or if an old mole is changing color or shape. Skin cancer is becoming much more common, and the incidence of melanoma, the most dangerous and life-threatening form of skin cancer, has risen in young adults nearly 1000 fold in the last 20 years. These new skin growths are the most important signal I have listed. What do they mean nutritionally? Moles and brown spots indicate disturbed antioxidant function, with deficiencies of selenium, vitamin E, vitamin C, and beta carotene, and glutathione being most important (see Chapter 6). Skin tags are associated with severe blood sugar disturbances (hypoglycemia) and being a form of skin "tumor", may indicate the existence of excessive cell growth (i.e. precancerous lesions). Do not get overly concerned. Skin tags which you have had for years that remain unchanged are relatively harmless. Be more concerned about newly developing ones. In these cases, you may be deficient in antioxidants. In addition, the organs controlling your blood sugar metabolism are malfunctioning (i.e. the pancreas, liver, and adrenal glands).

Brownish lesions which are raised are usually a form of skin tumor. Most often they are non-malignant. Yet they do indicate that a disturbance in your anti-cancer mechanisms exists. It is likely that your immune system is sluggish and that there are not enough protective nutrients to go around.

In summary, skin tags indicate blood sugar problems, chromium deficiency, and a lack of antioxidant nutrients. New or changing moles indicate a profound need for antioxidants and anti-cancer nutrients such as selenium, vitamin E, vitamin A, beta carotene, vitamin C, and garlic.

Garlic's high selenium and sulfur content assist the body in the synthesis of an enzyme known as glutathione peroxidase, discussed in more depth in Chapter 6. I have seen moles disappear upon adding selenium and garlic to the diet.

Melanomas are a more serious condition. However, nutrition is the most important element in their treatment. Melanomas can be dissolved with a cream rich in a special form of vitamin B-6 (known as *pyridoxal-5-phosphate*). Colorado researchers have discovered that topical application of vitamin E also helps. Megadoses of *natural* beta carotene, vitamin E, and vitamin C as well as at least 1 milligram of selenium are often necessary. I do not recommend self-treatment of any of these lesions, but I do believe you should find a physician who is open-minded enough to support any treatment you desire. After all, it is your body. You have the right to seek whatever treatment you desire.

#19 Easy bruising can mean a variety of things. First, it signals a deficiency of vitamin C and bioflavonoids. Bioflavonoids are a family of natural chemicals found primarily in fruits and vegetables, although many herbs are rich in them. In citrus fruits, bioflavonoids are concentrated primarily in the rind. Thus, eating the inner rinds of citrus fruits may prove helpful.

Bioflavonoids act by strengthening the inner lining of the blood vessel walls. Bruising also may be caused by a problem with liver function. A variety of blood clotting factors are synthesized in the liver. If it is malfunctioning, blood vessels will become weakened and bruising results. In this case, you will notice bruises without any obvious trauma.

The intestines serve as the primary source of vitamin K, where it is synthesized by intestinal bacteria. Vitamin K is needed for blood to clot normally. If you bruise easily, you may have a vitamin K deficiency secondary to the overgrowth of organisms such as yeasts in the intestines, which crowd out the useful bacteria. Thus, easy bruising may be an end result of using too many antibiotics. Antibiotics destroy the naturally occurring microbes in the bowel. These helpful microbes are then replaced by organisms which serve no useful function and actually steal rather than provide nutrients. The diet may predispose to this problem. Eating sugar and other refined carbohydrates encourages the growth of excessive amounts of yeasts in the bowel.

People who were not breast-fed will tend to have less of the helpful intestinal bacteria. These delicate, microbial creatures are known as *lactobacillus acidophilus* and *bifidus*. The bifidus bacteria are particularly vulnerable, and can easily be destroyed by such things as toxins in the environment, chlorine in the water, and, of course, antibiotics. The reason I am mentioning this is that many societies get extra acidophilus and bifidus bacteria in their diet. In general, Americans do not. Strong concoctions of fermented milk products rich in these bacteria form a regular part of the diet of Ukranians, Rumanians, Hungarians, Russians, Armenians, Lebanese, etc. Thus, these people are continually rebuilding their intestinal flora, plus they do not take antibiotics!

#20 Bleeding gums are also an indication of vitamin C and bioflavonoid deficiencies. However, they are a signal of a number of other problems as well, such as folic acid deficiency, intestinal infection, poor immunity, and infection within the gums themselves. A deficiency of a special nutrient known as *coenzyme Q-10* can also lead to gum disease. While not technically listed as a vitamin or mineral, coenzyme Q-10 is critically important for proper functioning of gum tissue and many other cells and organs.

#21 The existence of age spots means the body is undergoing a process known medically as *lipid peroxidation*. Be concerned if you are noticing an increase in the number or size of these spots. This means the fatty acids in your body are decomposing at a rapid rate and that you are susceptible to a variety of degenerative diseases including cancer.

Peroxides are fatty acids which have undergone a process known as *oxidation*. A good example of this is butter that is heated excessively. Butter is easily oxidized when heated and you will notice this if it turns dark brown. This is, in a sense, what happens in the body when fatty acids lining the membranes of your cells become "oxidized." In the case of living tissue, heat is not the factor initiating the oxidative changes. Brown spots are caused by radiation, toxic chemicals, toxic oils, and poor diet low in antioxidants, all of which initiate the oxidation of tissue fats. It has now been proven that the body's lipids degenerate more rapidly if deficiencies of selenium, vitamin E, beta carotene, vitamin C, pantothenic acid, and vitamin B-6 exist. A word of caution: poor quality fatty acids are worse for you than no fatty acids at all. Eating oils which are overheated (including butter), deep fried foods, highly processed fats such as commercial vegetable oils, margarine and lard only leads to an increase in the rate at which the fatty acids in our bodies degenerate (see Chapter 5). Anything which so greatly affects our cell membranes, the guardian and protector of the cells, will also increase your risks of degenerative disease, infection, and/or cancer.

The degeneration of our fatty acid coating, whether it be the skin, or the outer membrane of, say a liver cell, is one of the major factors predisposing us to cancer and immune decline. Avoid all substances which cause lipid peroxidation (see Chapter 6).

SOME SERIOUS WARNINGS

If you have any of the symptoms mentioned below, your body is trying to tell you something vital. If you don't become more aware and make some changes in the way you live, your life could be in danger! Here they are:

1. chest pain, worse upon exertion

2. severe leg pains or cramps which worsen when you exercise or walk

3. a noticeable decrease in memory or mental sharpness

4. moles which are growing in size or number

5. a noticeable decline in how fast your wounds heal

6. increased sensitivity to cold, noises, or smells

7. lowered resistance to colds or flu

8. poor or slow recovery from illness.

Not all of these symptoms indicate that a life-threatening problem exists. However, it is important to recognize them, if they occur, and correct the underlying causes before more serious problems arise. Most of these symptoms are a warning that there is a decline in the function of the immune, endocrine (i.e. hormonal), and circulatory systems.

CHAPTER 5
Avoiding The Time-Bombs

W hat are Time-Bombs? They are those substances found in our diet which have a potentially devastating effect upon the human body. Here is a list of the major Time-Bombs:

1) refined sugar

2) white flour

3) alcoholic beverages

4) processed or cured meats

5) deep-fried foods

6) refined vegetable oils, such as corn, sunflower, safflower and soybean oil

7) margarine and other hydrogenated vegetable oils, such as Crisco or shortening

8) pesticides and herbicides

9) industrial chemicals

10) radioactive chemicals

11) heavy metals

12) cigarettes

Are you scared? You should be, because each day you are getting a dose of not one but many of these Time-Bombs. However, there is no need to despair. Though it is not possible to entirely avoid exposure to these substances, you can largely control the first seven listed above. If you do nothing more than remove these seven dietary Time-Bombs from your lifestyle, you will enjoy better health.

The first seven items on the Time-Bomb list can be largely controlled by dietary and life style alterations. In this Chapter, I have concentrated primarily on five of these: item #1 (refined sugar), item #4 (processed and cured meats) and items #5, 6 & 7 (deep-fried foods, refined vegetable oils, margarine and other hydrogenated fats). Let's see how much exposure YOU are getting.

YOUR REFINED SUGAR TIME-BOMB QUOTIENT

Is sugar sweet or sour? I say it is sour. By definition, refined sugar includes white sugar, table sugar, brown sugar, corn syrup, malt syrup, glucose, molasses, and dextrose. Most of the refined sugar intake in the U.S.A. is in the form of white sugar. Refined sugar has many negative effects and no positive ones. Its consumption is associated with an increased incidence of diabetes, heart disease, cancer, high blood pressure and many other maladies. Even a little bit may be too much for your body to handle. As little as a teaspoonful per day can be harmful. Just think about the damage being done to those who are consuming it by the handful! You can find out your sugar quotient by taking the following test.

Circle the appropriate response. On the average, do you consume:

POINTS

1. DOUGHNUTS, CUPCAKES, AND/OR SWEETROLLS

1-2 per week 5

3-5 per week 10

1 per day. 15

2 or more per day. 20

2. CAKES, PIES, AND/OR BROWNIES

1-2 pieces per week. 5

3-5 pieces per week. 10

1 piece per day 15

2 or more pieces per day 20

3. POP (SWEETENED)

1 twelve oz. drink per week 5

2-5 twelve oz. drinks per week..............................10

1 twelve oz. drink per day 15

2 or more twelve oz. drinks per day 25

4. COFFEE OR TEA (SUGAR ADDED)

1-2 added teaspoons per week................................5

3-5 added teaspoons per week 10

1-3 added teaspoons per day 15

4 or more added teaspoons per day 20

5. OTHER SUGAR SWEETENED DRINKS
(KOOL-AID, HI-C, etc.)

1-2 drinks per week 5

3-4 drinks per week 10

1 drink per day...15

2 or more drinks per day 20

6. CANDY BARS

1 per week 5

2-3 per week 10

1 per day...15

2 or more per day...25

7. COOKIES

1-2 per week 5

3-4 per week 10

1 per day...15

2 or more per day...20

8. HARD CANDIES AND CHOCOLATES

2-5 pieces per week 5

1 piece per day 10

2-3 pieces per day 15

4 or more pieces per day 20

9. CEREALS (SUGAR-SWEETENED)

1 bowl per week 5

2-5 bowls per week 10

1 bowl per day 15

2 or more bowls per day . . . . 20 points

10. SALAD DRESSINGS, KETCHUP AND/OR STEAK SAUCE

2-5 times per week 5

1-2 times per day 10

3 or more times per day 15

11. YOGURT (SWEETENED), WHIPPING CREAM AND/OR NON-DAIRY CREAMER

1-4 times per week 5

once per day 10

2 or more times per day 15

12. CURED MEATS (bacon, ham, corned beef, bologna, hot dogs, etc.)

1-3 times per week 5

Once per day 10

2 or more times per day 15

13. ICE CREAM, MALTS, SHAKES, AND/OR SHERBET

1-2 servings per week 5

3-5 servings per week 10

1 serving per day 15

2 or more servings per day 20

YOUR SCORE _____

0-30 POINTS   You are consuming a small but significant amount of sugar. Cutting down on your sugar intake could lead to a noticeable improvement in your health.

35-70 POINTS   You are consuming sugar at a rate of a heaping teaspoon or more per day. It would be wise to slow down before the sugar slows *you* down.

75-130 POINTS   You are consuming sugar by the tablespoonful. Damage is being done. Curtail this excessive sugar intake immediately!

135-ABOVE   You are eating sugar every day by the handful. Wake up and realize the damage you are doing to yourself. You are in the category of consuming 100 to 200 pounds of sugar a year! Keep it up and you will likely develop diabetes, high blood pressure, heart disease, or cancer. Stop now, and you will recover much of your health.

Anyone with a score of 75 and above is living in the danger zone. At this level of sugar intake, there is a risk of damaging or even destroying the adrenal and thyroid glands. These delicate glands must work overtime to help the body deal with the excess sugar. After awhile under the pressure of constant bombardment of refined sugar, these glands literally burn out. To be sure, the glands are capable of regenerating and their function can return *if you make the appropriate dietary changes and get off the sugar*. There is a risk for permanent damage if you continue your sugar consumption. The more sugar consumed over the years, the more likely it is that you will have burned out a portion of your adrenal and thyroid glands. The following case history is an example of how this happens:

Mr. M was a long-standing lover of sweets. He not only ate them on a daily basis, but also gave various sweets such as cheesecake, chocolates, and candies to all of his friends. Needless to say, Mr. M is a sweet man. Although Mr. M presented with the primary complaint of angina and hardening of the arteries, his underlying problem was an *adrenal insufficiency* secondary to his sugar-ladened diet. Interestingly, his heart trouble improved (as did his weight) when he was placed on a diet free of all refined sugar. However, he continued to buy chocolates for his "friends" including his doctor who graciously received them, but secretly disposed of them in the trash can!

YOUR HYDROGENATED FAT TIME-BOMB QUOTIENT

Possibly the most common overall deficiency in this country is that of the essential fatty acids. These fatty acids are just as the term suggests — they are essential to life itself. In the typical American diet, these fats are being displaced by less useful ones, particularly hydrogenated fats, as you will find out by taking this exam.

Circle the correct response. On the average, do you consume:

1. **DEEP FRIED FOODS (French fries, fried chicken, fish sticks, potato chips, corn chips, etc.)**

   1-2 times per week 5

   3-4 times per week 10

   Once per day 15

   2 or more times per day 25

2. **BAKERY COOKED WITH SHORTENING (cookies, pies, pastries, cakes, etc.)**

   1-2 times per week 5

   3-4 times per week 10

   Once per day 15

   2 or more times per day 20

3. **MARGARINE (USED AS A SPREAD OR IN COOKING)**

   1-2 servings (tablespoons) per week 5

   3-6 servings per week 10

   1-2 servings per day 15

   3 or more servings per day 25

4. **CRACKERS OR SNACKS CONTAINING HYDROGENATED OR PARTIALLY HYDROGENATED OILS, LARD, OR SHORTENING**

   1-2 servings per week 5

   3-5 servings per week 10

   1-2 servings per day 15

   3 or more servings per day 20

5. **BREADS OR BUNS CONTAINING HYDROGENATED OR PARTIALLY HYDROGENATED OILS, LARD, OR SHORTENING**

   2-5 servings per week 5

   1 serving per day 10

   2-3 servings per day 15

   4 or more servings per day 20

6. **IMITATION ICE CREAM, WHIPPING CREAM, NON-DAIRY CREAMERS, AND VARIOUS COATED ICE-CREAM BARS**

   1-2 servings per week 5

   3-4 servings per week 10

   1-2 times per day 15

   3 or more servings per day 20

7. **CANDY BARS, CHOCOLATES, AND HARD CANDIES**

   1-2 servings per week 5

   3-4 servings per week 10

   1 serving per day 15

   2 or more servings per day 20

8. **FROZEN OR PACKAGED DINNERS, PIZZAS, FRENCH FRIES AND/OR TATER TOTS**

   1-3 times per week 5

   4-6 times per week 10

   1-2 times per day 15

   3 or more times per day. 20

9. **MAYONNAISE AND FOODS MADE WITH MAYONNAISE (potato salad, cole slaw, etc.)**

   1-3 times per week 5

   4-6 times per week 10

   1-2 times per day . . . . 15 points

   3 or more times per day. 20

   YOUR SCORE _____

0-30 POINTS   You are getting a small but significant amount of hydrogenated or harmful fats in your diet. Avoid the foods you are eating which contain these fats.

35-70 POINTS   You are eating harmful fats by the teaspoonful. These hydrogenated fats are harming you, your cells and your immune system. Avoid all foods containing these fats.

75-115 POINTS   You are eating harmful fats by the tablespoonful. Significant damage to your immune system is likely if you continue. Curtail your consumption of these noxious, hydrogenated fats immediately.

120 AND ABOVE — DANGER ZONE! You are eating hydrogenated fats by the tubfull! Your risk for developing heart disease, cancer, or some other life-threatening disease is quite high. It is crucial that you change your diet immediately. To help heal the damage, it is necessary to eat foods rich in natural, essential fatty acids and take fatty acid supplements.

HOW MARGARINE AND HYDROGENATED FATS ORIGINATED

The production of margarine was the result of a food shortage. During World War II, butter was scarce. Chemists experimented to find an alternative. They found that liquid vegetable oils could be turned into solid fat through a process known as *hydrogenation*. During this process, hydrogen gas is bubbled into the oil, which is heated to a high temperature. Nickel is then added to catalyze (speed up) the reaction. These hydrogenated fats are what make up margarine and shortening. In addition, in an attempt to mimic butter, synthetic dyes are added to turn the whitish-colored hydrogenated fats into margarine.

If you give it some thought, I think you will be able to understand how unnatural and unhealthy hydrogenated fats really are. True, margarine is touted as being low in cholesterol and saturated fats. Yet, it is high in unnatural fats, harmful fats and cancer-causing chemicals!

IS THERE A SAFE AMOUNT?

Even a small amount of hydrogenated fats and oils is too much. I recommend that hardened fats be eliminated entirely from the diet. Butter, of course, is an exception since it is natural and unaltered in its chemistry. However, one problem with butter is that it may contain Butter Yellow, a cancer-causing dye.

Even the typical liquid vegetable oils found in the supermarket must be used sparingly, if at all. Their use has been proven by research to be associated with an increased risk for developing cancer.

WHY PROCESSED FATS ARE SO BAD

If you are getting the wrong kinds of fats in your diet, beware. No doubt, your body needs a certain amount of fat every day, but it needs the "good" fats. If all you get is the processed kind, your body has no choice but to make use of them. Processed fats, especially the hydrogenated variety, confuse the body because their chemical structure is different than the naturally occurring fats normally recognized and utilized by the body.

Once the "bad" fats are absorbed, they are taken to the liver where they are stored or converted into energy. The chemistry of these fats is abnormal so the liver has a hard time trying to figure out what to do with them. When a cell is damaged and needs fatty acids for repair or other purposes, these abnormal fats will be made available to the cell, especially if there is a lack of natural, essential fats. The cell will attempt to place the abnormal fat into its membrane, resulting in a weakened, malfunctioning cell.

HAVE YOUR CELLS BECOME "HYDROGENATED"?

Would you believe that in all probability, you are "partially hydrogenated?" Over the years you have developed untold thousands of hardened (hydrogenated) cells. This is because these cells have inserted into their membranes trans fats from a dose of margarine or from some French fries cooked in a deep fryer, etc.

An example of this is what happens to white blood cells. These cells incorporate the hydrogenated fats you eat into their membranes. When this happens, the white cells become sluggish in function, and their membranes actually become stiff! Such white blood cells are poor defenders against infection. This leaves the body wide open to all sorts of derangements of the immune system. Cancer, or infections by yeasts, bacteria and viruses can more easily take a foothold.

Chemically altered and hydrogenated fats are no longer a food. They, in effect, become a poison, polluting the body's cells and organs. Once deposited within the tissues, these fats damage the cells and organs

In fact, one of the quickest ways to paralyze your immune system is to eat, on a daily basis, significant quantities of deep fried foods, or fats such as margarine, partially hydrogenated cottonseed/palm/corn/ or sunflower oil, or lard.

HOW FATS BECOME HYDROGENATED (THE TRANS FATTY ACID STORY)

Trans fats result from the chemical process of hydrogenation. As described previously, chemists take oils such as corn, cottonseed, and safflower which are normally liquid at room temperature and heat them to a very high temperature. They then add chemicals including the metal nickel to cause a kinking in the oils' molecular bonds. This causes the chemical structure to be altered from the normal *cis* configuration to the *trans* structure. These trans fatty acids are *not found in nature*. Thus, man is unable to properly utilize them. In effect, what was once a food, i.e. liquid vegetable oils, has now been turned into a laboratory aberration — a freak, but not an accidental one!

All this is done for effect. Marketability, shelf life, and consumer appeal are the goals of the hydrogenated fat industry. These fats have a forever shelf life. Yet, your life may be shelved if you continue to eat them. While hydrogenated fats may not become rancid on the shelf, they induce all sorts of rancidity problems within the body. They waste antioxidants such as vitamin E and selenium which function to prevent fats from becoming rancid.

No wonder that a high consumption of margarine, shortening, and other hydrogenated fats is associated with a greater incidence of a variety of cancers. A list of conditions and diseases associated with their consumption includes:

1. Alzheimer's Disease

2. Atherosclerosis

3. Autoimmune Diseases

4. Cancer

5. Chronic Candidiasis

6. Diabetes

7. Eczema

8. Heart Disease

9. High Blood Pressure

10. Parkinson's Disease

11. PMS

12. Psoriasis

Avoid hydrogenated fats like you would avoid the plague.

DR. IGRAM'S FIVE SIMPLE RULES FOR AVOIDING HYDROGENATED FATS

1. Shop in the outer aisles at your grocery store. Fresh foods, fruits, vegetables, fresh meats, eggs, milk, and cheese do not contain added oils.

2. Use only extra virgin olive oil or butter in cooking or food preparation. Other cold-pressed vegetable oils are acceptable, particularly cold-pressed sesame, peanut, walnut and avocado oils.

3. Always ask your server what the restaurant is sauteeing the food in. Most restaurants carry olive oil or will carry it upon demand. If you forget to ask, *odds are the food will be cooked with margarine or hydrogenated fats.*

4. Tell your server as soon as you see him/her to hold the bread basket. This way your hunger will not overwhelm you. Most crackers and rolls contain hydrogenated fats.

5. Read all labels on canned, bottled, or packaged foods purchased at the grocery store. If you see the words hydrogenated, partially hydrogenated, or shortening, do not buy it.

WHAT ARE THE GOOD FATS?

I would be doing you a major disservice if I only told you which fats to avoid. Fats and oils have been used in food preparation for centuries. Olive oil is probably the most ancient cooking oil, used as far back as ancient Egyptian times. Olive oil has proven itself with the test of time. Yet, only in the last decade has modern medical science recognized its healthful benefits. Another oil which has been used for centuries is flax seed oil. This is also known as linseed oil (food-grade). Europeans have extolled its health benefits since the Middle Ages.

The Eskimos' high fat diet has been very beneficial to their health. Although Eskimos eat lots of fat, they eat natural fats, primarily from fish, whale, and seal oils. Thus, they do not have the problems we do from eating altered or unnatural ones.

No doubt the oils of certain seeds such as safflower and sunflower seeds have healthy components. Yet, these oils are beneficial only if they are extracted from the seeds under the appropriate conditions. The only way to insure the nutritional value of these oils is to extract them by cold-pressing, without the use of heat or chemicals. All the typical vegetable oils in the supermarket are extracted under conditions of very high temperatures and with the use of chemicals. This process upsets the chemistry of the oils, and destroys the naturally occurring antioxidants. For example, sunflower oil naturally contains lots of vitamin E, the major antioxidant found in fats and oils. However, when sunflower oil is heat-extracted, all the vitamin E is destroyed. This is why food processors have to add synthetic antioxidants, such as BHT to their oils. BHT is a known carcinogen.

Most truly cold-pressed oils can be discerned by a simple fact: they have a sediment at the bottom of the bottle. Extra-virgin olive oil, while cold-pressed, does not usually contain a sediment. Most of the content of the olive is made up of oils. Olives as a food, are one of the richest food sources of vegetable oil. Olive oil is highly beneficial. It does not become rancid easily and can be heated to higher temperatures than other vegetable oils without being damaged. Olive oil has beneficial effects upon the circulation, reducing cholesterol levels and improving blood flow. In addition, it is highly digestible. I recommend olive oil as the major cooking oil you should use.

Butter can be used in cooking, but low heat should be used. Clarified butter is the best cooking butter, since it can withstand higher temperatures.* At moderately high cooking temperatures, the fatty acids in regular butter are damaged. If heated excessively, it becomes rancid and toxic. If you burn the butter, don't use it. Reduce the temperature and start all over again.

Cold-pressed corn, sunflower, safflower, almond, walnut, avocado, peanut, and sesame oils can also be used in cooking. Be careful not to heat them excessively. Most of these are higher than olive oil or butter in polyunsaturated oils. Excessive heating damages the polyunsaturated oils, causing them to be toxic and potentially cancer-promoting.

WHAT FOODS ARE RICH IN ESSENTIAL FATTY ACIDS

Only a few common foods are naturally rich in essential fatty acids. A partial list of them includes:

1. avocado
2. almonds
3. beans
4. brazil nuts
5. eggs
6. fish
7. mustard seeds
8. pecans
9. pine nuts
10. poppy seeds
11. pumpkin seeds
12. rice germ or bran
13. soy beans
14. sunflower seeds

* See recipe in recipe section (Part II) of this book.

15. walnuts

16. wheat germ

17. wild game

Wild game is the richest meat source of essential fatty acids. This is due to the fatty acid-rich diet of these animals. I highly recommend the addition of game such as pheasant, quail, deer, elk, duck and goose to your diet.

WHAT ABOUT ESSENTIAL FATTY ACID SUPPLEMENTS?

I believe firmly in the use of nutritional supplements. No area deserves more attention than the need to supplement our diet with essential fatty acids.

Essential fatty acids, by the strictest definition, are those fats which cannot be made in the body and must be consumed via the diet. Only two such fatty acids exist, namely, *linoleic* and *linolenic* acid. Excellent supplemental sources of these fatty acids include flax seed, evening primrose, sunflower, and safflower oil. Other rich sources are sesame, corn, wheat germ, cod liver, almond, walnut, and soy bean oil.*

Note: Olive oil contains only small quantities of the essential fatty acids. However, it contains a number of other useful oils, such as *oleic acid.*

For correcting deficiencies, I prefer the use of flax seed and primrose oil. A great deal of research has been done on the therapeutic benefits of these oils. In addition, both contain appreciable quantities of the rarer linolenic acid, while containing less linoleic acid than the other oils. Deficiency of linoleic acid is less common since oils rich in it such as corn, sunflower, and safflower are more prevalent in our diets.

A deficiency of essential fatty acids can be caused by a variety of factors including:

1. alcohol consumption

2. antibiotic overuse

3. chewing tobacco

4. cigarette smoking

5. excess dietary hydrogenated, partially hydrogenated, and deep-fried fats (the #1 cause in America today)

6. high intake of saturated fats

7. high sugar intake (the #2 cause)

* Make sure you use these oils only if they are cold-pressed.

8. intestinal fungal or yeast infection

9. severe. prolonged emotional stress

10. toxic chemical exposure

11. zinc. magnesium. vitamin C. vitamin B-6. niacin. or biotin deficiency

Diseases caused by or related to essential fatty acid deficiency include:

1. Adrenal insufficiency

2. Allergies

3. Atherosclerosis

4. Atopy

5. Chron's disease

6. Diabetes

7. Eczema and psoriasis

8. Hypothyroidism

9. Ulcerative colitis

THE ATOPIC INDIVIDUAL

A good example to help point out how severe health problems can be caused by essential fatty acid deficiency is *atopy*. This term relates to how certain persons inherit defective genes from their mothers. fathers. or grandparents. The defect lies in an inability to make proper use of essential fatty acids. These atopic individuals are quite vulnerable to asthma. hayfever. food allergies. sinus problems. and PMS. They are also far more susceptible to the ill-effects of consuming processed or hydrogenated oils.

It has been shown that the symptoms and illnesses associated with the atopic state improve with fatty acid supplementation. A generous supply of vitamins and minerals. especially zinc. magnesium. vitamin B-6. and biotin also help.

Most people with atopic sensitivity have a condition known as the "toxic" colon. Often. a history of constipation and hardened stools is elicited. The overgrowth of yeasts and "unfriendly" bacteria in the colon helps maintain the constipation and toxic state. Supplementation with essential fatty acids often helps relieve the constipation and, thereby, improve colon toxicity.

Numerous other symptoms may signal essential fatty acid deficiency including:

1. bleeding gums

2. brittle hair or nails

3. cold extremities

4. dryness of skin behind the ears

5. dry or flaky skin

6. dry or oily hair

7. dry patches of skin on the face

8. excess thirst

9. excess oil on the face or hair

10. excess or lack of ear wax

11. hair loss

12. itchy ears

13. irritable or sluggish bowels

14. lowered resistence to infection

15. poor wound healing

16. slow-growing hair or nails

17. yeast infections

IMMUNE BREAKDOWN:
A CONSEQUENCE OF ESSENTIAL FATTY ACID DEFICIENCY

No doubt, essential fatty acid deficiency can result in a wide range of symptoms as you can see from the above. Let's concentrate on symptoms 14, 15, and 17 — symptoms indicating poor immune function. The immune system needs essential fatty acids. It cannot function properly without them. Every immune cell and organ in the body needs a daily supply to stay in optimal working order. And these cells and organs will degenerate unless they get an adequate supply of essential fatty acids. This condition is known as *cellular atrophy*.

THE SKIN: OUR FIRST LINE OF DEFENSE

Essential fatty acids are necessary for maintaining the structural integrity of every cell and cell membrane in the body. The skin is the first defense against invasion by microbes. What is it that keeps the skin taut and free of cracks, wounds and cuts? Primarily, the essential fatty acids. These fatty acids are also required to help seal any cuts or wounds that do occur. Tiny tears in our skin occur every day, although you may not be able to see them. The body heals these tears by mobilizing extra fatty acids from the liver and any that are stored in body fat. In addition, zinc, selenium and several B-vitamins are required to help in the utilization of these fatty acids.

Fatty acids on and within our skin also protect us by having direct, toxic effects on any harmful microorganisms. They are truly our skin's natural antibiotics.

There is, however, a more insideous effect of this deficiency upon our immune system — damage to the cell membrane. Several nutrients are needed to keep cell membranes healthy. The list includes selenium, vitamin E, vitamin A, cholesterol (believe it or not, cholesterol has many useful functions), and essential fatty acids. If the cell membrane is not supplied with an adequate amount of any one or all of these nutrients, it will break down. Obviously, if the membranes of immune cells such as white blood cells and lymphocytes begin to break apart, all kinds of problems will result. The body is left wide open to infection by all sorts of microbes, not to mention cancer.

Do you know how much surface would be covered if all 70 trillion of your cell membranes were flattened out, end to end? They would cover an area the size of Texas or better! This certainly gives you an idea of how important proper nutrition is. Remember, years of abuse caused by eating the wrong kind of fats is not corrected overnight. It may take weeks or months to solve the problem.

YOUR PROCESSED/CURED MEAT TIME-BOMB QUOTIENT

Meats can be good for you, that is, if they are fresh or if they do not contain chemicals, hormones, pesticides, preservatives, or other additives. *Processed* meats, that is meats cured with nitrates, are a poor choice especially when fresh meats are so readily available. Cured meats are loaded with chemical preservatives (nitrates, BHT, BHA), coloring agents, sugar, and other sweeteners such as dextrose and corn syrup. Take this test to find out how much exposure *you* are getting:

Circle the correct response. On the average, do you consume:

1. HOT DOGS AND/OR WIENERS

1 per week .... 5 points

2-3 per week .... 10 points

4-6 per week .... 15 points

1 or more daily..................................... 25 points

2. HAM AND/OR SPAM

1 serving per week .... 5 points

2-3 servings per week .... 10 points

4-6 servings per week .... 15 points

1 or more servings daily............................ 20 points

3. PASTRAMI, CHIPPED BEEF, AND/OR CORNED BEEF

1 serving per week .... 5 points

2-3 servings per week .... 10 points

4-6 servings per week .... 15 points

1 or more servings daily............................ 20 points

4. BOLOGNA, SALAMI, AND/OR OTHER DELI LUNCHEON MEATS

1 serving per week .... 5 points

2-3 servings per week .... 10 points

4-6 servings per week .... 15 points

1 or more servings daily............................ 20 points

5. SAUSAGES AND/OR BRATWURST

1 serving per week .... 5 points

2-3 servings per week .... 10 points

4-6 servings per week .... 15 points

1 serving per day .... 20 points

2 or more servings per day.......................... 25 points

6. TURKEY HAM, TURKEY SALAMI, AND/OR TURKEY PASTRAMI

1-3 servings per week .... 5 points
4-6 servings per week .... 10 points
1 or more servings daily............................. 15 points

7. BACON AND/OR BREAKFAST STRIPS

1-2 slices per week .... 5 points
3-6 slices per week .... 10 points
1 slice per day...................................... 15 points
2-3 slices per day .... 20 points
4 or more slices per day .... 25 points

8. BEEF JERKEY

1-2 sticks per week .... 5 points
3-4 sticks per week .... 10 points
5-6 sticks per week .... 15 points
1 or more sticks daily............................... 20 points

9. PORK AND BEANS, OR SIMILAR CANNED PORK PRODUCTS

1-3 servings per week .... 5 points
4-6 servings per week .... 10 points
1-2 servings daily .... 15 points
3 or more servings daily............................. 20 points

YOUR SCORE _____

0-15 POINTS You are doing well. Considering how available and common these meats are, it is remarkable that your exposure is so minimal. However, eliminating these meats entirely would help your overall health. "Zero" points is certainly what you should strive for.

20-45 POINTS Each week you are getting a significant dose of nitrates from eating processed meats. The nitrates in meats and the other ingredients, such as coloring agents, sugar, etc. are bad for you. At this time you may not notice any ill effects from eating these meats But eventually, it will catch up with you and have a negative bearing on your health.

50-80 POINTS It appears that you are getting a daily dose of nitrated and/or processed meats. This is dangerous. Nitrates are curing agents, acting to retard spoilage of the meat. In order for them to be effective, they need to be added to the food in rather large amounts. At this level of exposure, it is likely that you are experiencing at least two ill effects from the nitrates: 1) digestive disturbances, and 2) fatigue. The fatigue is caused by an interesting mechanism. Nitrates combine with hemoglobin in the blood and turn it into its inactive form. This is known medically as *methemoglobin*. Methemoglobin is useless to the body, since it cannot carry oxygen to the cells. The transport of oxygen is the primary function of the normal hemoglobin molecule. This lack of oxygen disrupts the cells' metabolism, resulting in symptoms ranging from fatigue to poor circulation and headaches.

85-115 POINTS You are eating nitrated and/or processed meats on a daily basis. Curtail your intake of these meats before they cause you to be curtailed! If you continue, you may end up just like the animals from which they are made — belly up! I am serious. Eating these foods in this quantity is damaging, leading to problems such as allergies, immune system disorders, and even heart disease, heart attacks, and cancer. Cancer is the most ominous result. Nitrates combine in the stomach with proteins to form substances known as *nitrosamines*. Nitrosamines are proven carcinogens. They irritate the cells lining the stomach and intestines, causing inflammation. Nitrosamines interact with the genes of these cells causing them to change over to cancerous cells.

The reduction in blood flow and blood oxygen content are why, in part, nitrates aggravate the heart, increasing heart-related symptoms. It is my contention that many a heart attack has been brought on by eating nitrate-laden meats.

120-ABOVE You are eating an unbelievably large amount of nitrated and processed meats. Trouble is forthcoming if it hasn't already occurred. These meats and the chemicals they contain are, without doubt, damaging the lining of your stomach and intestines. They are depressing your immune system and predisposing you to cancer of the digestive tract and possibly cancer of other organs as well. The liver, the body's factory for detoxifying noxious agents, is no doubt being worn down by the extra burden of additives and chemicals.

This much exposure to nitrates through eating the previously mentioned meats greatly increases cancer risks. Heed this warning seriously! Remove all these meats from your diet, and when you eat meat, buy fresh meats such as hamburger, steaks, or chops.

If you do have health problems, they are most likely related to the consumption of processed meats. This will be confirmed by your increased sense of well-being and the improvement in energy you will experience when they are eliminated from your diet.

The damaging effects of nitrates and nitrosamines can best be described by the renowned cancer researcher, Kedar Prasad, Ph.D., who states: *"Nitrosamines, which result from the nitrosation of food constituents by ingested nitrites or nitrates, are one of the most potent human carcinogens."* He also states that the largest source of nitrite intake in the U.S.A. is from cured meats, although cigarette smoke is the primary source of direct exposure to nitrosamines.

Plenty of evidence exists that a high intake of or exposure to nitrates, nitrites, and nitrosamines initiates changes in the body which may ultimately lead to cancer. The organs most heavily hit are the esophagus, stomach, large intestine, bladder, and lungs. Yet, they may also cause an even more sinister disease as is illustrated by this case history:

A two-year-old girl developed a variety of symptoms for which the cause was unknown. Initially, tests were performed but no diagnosis was determined. The illness began taking a new course — she developed an enlarged, malfunctioning heart. The best of medical minds were having difficulty diagnosing the problem. Finally, an analysis was done on her diet, since the illness appeared to be similar to Keshan disease, a disease of the heart seen in certain children in China. Keshan disease is due to a selenium deficiency, a mineral whose importance is discussed at length in Chapter 6. Indeed, testing did show that she was selenium deficient. A diagnosis of selenium-deficient cardiomyopathy was established, a disease which leads to the degeneration of heart muscle. But even more important was the diet analysis. Her daily diet consisted of grits and sausage for breakfast, a hot dog with pork and beans for lunch, and pork and beans plus rice for dinner! Each of these meals contained a dose of nitrates. The only beverages she had were Kool-Aid and water. No wonder she was sick to her heart.

Most of us have eaten foods such as refined sugar, hydrogenated oils, and processed meats throughout our lives. Some have consumed them in larger quantities than others. All this is in the past. Now is the time for a better, healthier future. Much of the damage can be repaired by changing old habits, eating wholesome, health-giving foods, and taking special nutrients known as antioxidants, as you will see from the next chapter.

CHAPTER 6
Antioxidants To Your Rescue

If you are plagued with an illness such as diabetes, heart disease, high blood pressure, arthritis, lung disease, or any other disease of civilization, don't despair. There is a cure! Natural substances known as *antioxidants* can come to your rescue.

Most Americans are deficient in this key group of nutrients. Antioxidants can be defined just as the name indicates: they are anti (against) oxidation. Oxidation is a chemical reaction which normally occurs within the body. When oxidative reactions occur in excess, cell damage and even cellular death result. Antioxidants are useful since they stop abnormal oxidative reactions before the damage occurs.

An example of the process of oxidation with which you are familiar is what happens to a nail or any other piece of iron when exposed to the outdoors. The nail or iron becomes rusty (oxidized). This is because oxygen from the air freely combines with the iron. If left unprotected, a similar process can occur to the membranes (walls) of your cells. The fatty acids of the cell walls, the most vulnerable part of the cell, can actually become rancid as a result of the oxidative process.

Antioxidants shield our cells from damage due to a variety of noxious agents including toxins, radiation, carcinogens, and stress. In particular, antioxidants protect us from reactions within our bodies which generate *free radicals*. Free radicals are molecules which can damage our cells. Oxidation reactions and free radicals go hand in hand. They both occur within our bodies in response to stress.

47

Every day each of us forms millions of free radicals. Our ability to quench or destroy free radicals before they cause tissue damage is dependent upon an adequate supply of antioxidants. Vitamin E, vitamin A, vitamin C, pantothenic acid, beta carotene, coenzyme Q-10 and selenium are examples of natural antioxidants which block free radical reactions.

FOOD REFINEMENT: ITS EFFECT ON ANTIOXIDANTS

The current American diet is an antioxidant-depleted one. The refinement of food destroys approximately 90% of the naturally occurring antioxidants. Even worse, many of these refined foods go on to damage and destroy what few antioxidants there are left in the body. An example of this is margarine or refined vegetable oils. Both of these fats, which are common ingredients in processed, packaged foods, rapidly deplete the body's reserves of antioxidants. In particular, vegetable oils cause the consumption of vitamin E. I always advises those who consume refined oils to take at least an extra 800 I.U. of vitamin E daily. For the vitamin E to be most effective, it must be in the unbound state. These types of vitamin E molecules are known chemically as alpha-tocopherol or mixed tocopherols (see appendix B).

THE SELENIUM CONTROVERSY

Selenium is a mineral. It is one of the few minerals containing antioxidant properties. This is discussed in more detail in Chapter 8. For years there has been a debate about whether or not too much selenium is harmful. Thus, most nutritionists and doctors have been cautious in suggesting selenium supplements and have kept the dosages to a minimum. I would much rather see you have higher amounts of selenium than to get too little. Why? Because in those regions of the world with near toxic levels of selenium in their soil or water, there is little or no cancer! Selenium may well be the single most important antioxidant for preventing cancer. A nation with an incidence of one in three people contracting cancer should not worry about getting too much selenium. If you live in states with selenium depleted soils such as Wisconsin, Illinois, Indiana, Michigan, Ohio, Maine, New York, New Jersey, Pennsylvania, and Florida, you need to take selenium supplements. What is the best dosage? That depends on how much selenium you are getting in your food and water (see appendix A, chart #3). A good rule of thumb is to take at least 400 micrograms (mcgs.) per day as a preventive measure. People living in low selenium regions who are exposed to radiation, toxic chemicals or excessive amounts of sunlight, may need to increase this dosage.

CONDITIONS INCREASING THE NEED FOR ANTIOXIDANTS

There are several situations where the body's needs for antioxidant protection increases. I will discuss a few of the more common ones.

I. HEAVY METAL POLLUTION

Heavy metal pollution is real and has now hit disasterous proportions. Scientists are finding unbelievably high levels of lead, mercury, aluminum and cadmium within the soil and water. The end result is increased levels of these toxic metals within our bodies. Even the Eskimos living in the North Pole are affected. Scientists have discovered a three-fold increase of mercury in the Eskimos' hair over that of their ancestors 500 years ago. Even greater increases are seen with lead.

Heavy metals cause the consumption of antioxidants. People at risk for heavy metal poisoning include car mechanics, industrial workers, dentists, jewelers, painters, dialysis patients, road workers, and artists. Also included are those who have lived in a home with lead pipes or who have used aluminum cookware and/or antacids over a prolonged period. Extra doses of antioxidants are needed to block the ill-effects of heavy metal poisoning. Here is a chart to help guide you if you have a history of exposure.

1. Lead - take extra calcium, vitamin C, vitamin E and selenium.

2. Cadmium - take extra zinc (most important), vitamin C, and selenium.

3. Mercury - take extra selenium (most important) and vitamin C.

4. Aluminum - take extra selenium, vitamin C and vitamin E. Calcium and magnesium also help by blocking aluminum absorption.

5. Arsenic - take extra niacin, B-6, vitamin C and selenium.

II. AIR POLLUTION

It has been known for years that the pollutants we breath can damage our lungs. More recently, it has been found that this damage is mediated by free radical reactions and that antioxidants halt these reactions. Vitamin E, beta carotene, vitamin C, and folic acid are of particular value in protecting lung tissue from being damaged. Everyone living in areas such as Los Angeles where smog is a problem should take at least 75,000 I.U. of beta carotene, 1,200 I.U. of vitamin E, and 5 mgs. of folic acid. These dosages will protect the internal organs, particularly the lungs, from the ill-effects of air pollutants.

III. RADIATION

Exposure to radioactivity greatly increases the need for antioxidants. Many of the health problems induced by radiation could be prevented by taking antioxidants, especially beta carotene, vitamin E, and selenium. The effect is more powerful if the antioxidants are taken immediately before or after a radiation insult. We are all receiving increasing amounts of radiation. Those acutely exposed to radiation from x-rays, radiation leakage, ultraviolet rays, etc. would greatly benefit by adding these antioxidants to the diet.

It has also been discovered that radiation damage resulting from ultraviolet light can be blocked by certain B-vitamins, particularly pantothenic acid, PABA, and DMG (formerly known as vitamin B-15). PABA (para-amino benzoic acid) is a metabolic by-product of the B-vitamin folic acid. Large doses of folic acid, that is greater than 5 mgs. have also proven helpful.

SUPPLEMENTING YOUR DIET

Flooding your blood with extra levels of protective antioxidants is a smart move. Why? Because research is showing that most health problems are related to too little antioxidant protection. Cancer patients, for example, have significantly lower blood levels of vitamins A, C, E, folic acid, and beta carotene than do normal people. These nutrients are rapidly used up by the immune system in an attempt to battle the cancer. The same holds true for other degenerative diseases such as arthritis, emphysema, and heart disease. Most of us are getting too little antioxidant protection. It is not worth taking a chance. I believe you must take antioxidants in abundance.

I suppose some are worried about getting too much of a good thing. This is difficult to do since antioxidants are used up literally as fast as we can put them in! That's right. The intensity of the chemical reactions which cause diseases such as cancer and arthritis is so great that the antioxidants are used up almost as soon as you swallow them. Billions of molecules of vitamin E, beta carotene, and selenium are utilized every day by your liver alone to protect it from free radical damage. Without an adequate supply of these and other antioxidants, our tissues would age and degenerate very rapidly. In fact, this does occur in some extreme cases.

Stress can also cause premature aging. Stress causes the loss of several important nutrients including vitamins A, C, the B-vitamins, zinc, magnesium, and selenium. The body's reservoirs of pantothenic acid (vitamin B-5) are rapidly diminished during stressful episodes. This vitamin has a potent antioxidant function. It is also needed for the synthesis of adrenal hormones. If the stress is prolonged and the levels of pantothenic acid become too low, a relatively serious problem can result: adrenal exhaustion. Without pantothenic acid, cells within the adrenal glands begin to die, a process known as *atrophy*. Thus, adrenal hormone production drops dramatically. People who are under stress should take high doses of pantothenic acid, as much as 2 to 6 grams daily. The doses should be spread out over the day, with morning, mid-morning, afternoon and evening doses being the ideal.

BETA CAROTENE TO THE RESCUE

Beta carotene is an important factor in preventing cell and organ damage. In particular, it protects cells from the damaging effects of radiation. Beta carotene is found primarily in plants. Its function is to protect them from damage due to the sun's rays. Beta carotene plays a similar role in respect to human skin and is normally concentrated there in significant amounts. The value of this nutrient is so vast that an entire chapter could be devoted to it.

If you do not eat beta carotene-rich fruits and/or vegetables on a regular basis, it is likely that you are deficient in this important antioxidant.* If prolonged enough, a deficiency in beta carotene could be risky. With the acceleration of the current cancer rate and the infectious disease epidemic (AIDS, etc.) you are at a double risk. Beta carotene is of major importance in protecting the cell's nucleus from being damaged. Nuclear material, which includes the genes and chromosomes, is delicate and extremely vulnerable to the ill-effects of radioactive waves, ultraviolet light, synthetic chemicals, heavy metals and other noxious substances. This damage is more likely to occur when the immune system is under stress, since it is involved in the repair of damaged nuclear material.

Another reason why more beta carotene is needed is the loss of the ozone layer. Ozone is known mainly for its harmful effects. Yet, it has a protective function as well. The ozone layer in the upper reaches of the atmosphere screens out much of the potentially damaging ultraviolet waves from the sun. However, pollutants in the air, particularly substances known as *chloroflurocarbons,* destroy the ozone molecules. This has led to a measurable decrease in the levels of ozone in the atmosphere. With the depletion of the ozone layer, more ultraviolet waves are reaching us now than ever — enter beta carotene. If there is enough beta carotene in the skin, these waves are blocked before they can get into the body and cause damage.

For these and other reasons, I recommend that you double your consumption of beta carotene-rich foods. Modern man gets significantly less beta carotene in his diet than did his ancestors, yet his needs are greater!

* Foods rich in beta carotene include apricots, cantaloupe, papayas, mangoes, red peppers, hot peppers, winter squash, pumpkin, squash, sweet potatoes, carrots, and dark green leafy vegetables. Foods with less, but still valuable amounts, include watermelon, cabbage, oranges, tangerines, cherries, peaches, avocados, nectarines, and tomatoes.

YOUR DAILY FIX OF BETA CAROTENE

An easy way to get a daily dose of beta carotene is to eat some dried apricots. Get only the unsulfured variety, usually found in health food stores. Half a cantaloupe per day would help, and for those who do not have to watch their carbohydrate intake, a sweet potato a day could well keep the doctor away. I take an even easier fix. Every day I swallow anywhere between 20 to 50 tiny chlorella tablets.* Chlorella is one of the finest natural sources of beta carotene. The carotenes in chlorella help protect the digestive organs from cancer and pre-cancerous changes. In addition, these miraculous tablets pull out poisons which build up in the body and within the digestive tract.

Another source of beta carotene is the synthetic form found in multiple vitamins and in most beta carotene supplements. While less costly, its effects on the body are as cheap as its price. The antioxidant and protective ability of man-made beta carotene is inadequate. Several all-natural beta carotene supplements are now available. Natural beta carotene is an extract and is, therefore, more expensive than the synthetic. When it comes to your body, I advise against going second best. If it is difficult for you to get a daily dose of natural beta carotene from foods, I recommend that you take either chlorella or a natural beta carotene extract.**

THE BODY'S OWN ANTIOXIDANTS

There are two basic categories of antioxidants: those found within food sources, and those that are made within the body. Examples of the first type include vitamin E, beta carotene, vitamin A, and selenium.

The second type, those that can be synthesized in the body, includes coenzyme Q-10, glutathione, SOD (superoxide dismutase), catalase, and pantothenic acid. The body works hard to synthesize these antioxidants. However, before it can do so, it is necessary to supply the body with the raw materials needed for synthesis. For example, the antioxidant enzyme

* I prefer the cell-wall disintegrated Sun Chlorella brand made by YSK International (see appendix B). Their manufacturing process makes the beta carotene more available for absorption than other forms of chorella.

** A few companies have made available natural beta carotene supplements, which are extracted from algae. Premium-Grade beta carotene is an excellent choice. See appendix B for ordering information.

SOD which is found in every cell in the body cannot be made without amino acids (from proteins), as well zinc, copper, and manganese as raw materials. Before glutathione can be made, there must be enough protein in the diet, especially proteins rich in the amino acids methionine and cysteine. This includes primarily animal proteins such as milk, eggs, and meat. These internal or "home-made" antioxidants are every bit as important as the dietary ones. The two work together to protect the body from all sorts of harmful chemical reactions.

GLUTATHIONE INHIBITS AGING

Scientific evidence is accumulating that glutathione inhibits the aging process. Glutathione is the major antioxidant found within all animal cells. It is found in every creature from insects to man. Every day our bodies synthesize millions of glutathione molecules. In the last 20 years, volumes of research data points to glutathione as being the number one anti-aging substance. This is best summarized by the following facts:

1. Levels of glutathione decline with age, and are particularly low in those with premature aging.

2. People whose glutathione levels remain high are more free of diseases or sickness. In addition, tests show them to be biologically younger.

3. Animals fed substances needed for glutathione synthesis, such as methionine, cysteine, or selenium lived longer than those that were not supplemented.

A test is now available to determine the activity of glutathione (as glutathione peroxidase). For more information, see Part III, Section 3. Since glutathione peroxidase is probably the most crucial cancer-protective enzyme in the body, it is important that everyone have their glutathione activity assessed.

THE LIVER — OUR BODY'S ANTIOXIDANT FACTORY

The liver is the hub of all manufacturing activity within the body. This is where antioxidants such as SOD, catalase, coenzyme Q-10, and glutathione are made. Thousands of other important substances are also made in the liver. The liver is also the storehouse for most of the body's antioxidants. It is important to have a healthy liver in order to remain free of disease.

DON'T FORGET YOUR DAILY DOSE OF VITAMIN E

Vitamin E is not just for sexual vigor. It is the key antioxidant for protecting cell membranes. This is because the major constituent of cell membranes is fat. These fats include the essential fatty acids, cholesterol, and lecithin. Vitamin E itself is soluble in fat, which means it readily dissolves into cell membranes. By binding to the fatty acids of cell membranes, vitamin E directly stops the occurrence of reactions which would otherwise be damaging. It thus prevents these fatty substances from oxidizing. Such damage can and does lead to cell damage and/or death.

NASA AND THE VITAMIN E CONNECTION

A good example of cellular damage due to vitamin E deficiency is what happens to the red blood cells of astronauts. While in outer space, astronauts are exposed to dangerously high amounts of radiation from the sun. They have no earthly atmosphere to protect them from the sun's rays. The astronauts' red blood cells absorb some of this excess radiation, and the cell membranes break down. The result is a tired, sick astronaut! The fatigue they experience is somewhat like that seen in anemic people. Researchers at NASA found that vitamin E stopped this harmful reaction, and thus supplemented the astronauts' diet.

The useful functions of vitamin E are many. Conditions in which vitamin E has proven helpful include some forms of anemia, low HDL cholesterol (the "good" cholesterol), heart disease, arthritis, acne, diabetes, infertility, fibrocystic breast disease, Raynaud's disease, lupus, heart disease, and vasculitis (inflammation of the blood vessels). Vitamin E is not a miracle cure for these conditions, but if taken consistently in the proper form and dose, it usually helps.

THE RIGHT TYPE OF VITAMIN E

There are many types of vitamin E available on the market. What is the right form? Certain of these brands claim to be all-natural. However, natural vitamin E is often chemically altered. This process is called *esterification*. This type of vitamin E does not work as well as the crude, unaltered vitamin E extract. Synthetic vitamin E is far less potent than the natural. Some products labeled as "natural vitamin E" contain as little as 10% natural E, the rest being synthetic. Unfortunately, this type of labeling is not illegal. In addition, the proper dosage depends upon the condition being treated.

Are you totally confused? Don't be. Here are some simple rules to follow in selecting the appropriate vitamin E:

1. If your vitamin E is not working, there is probably no active vitamin E in your product. In other words, the vitamin E you are using is probably a sham.

2. Any vitamin E product (400 I.U.) that costs less than $8.00 per bottle is likely to be so much garbage. Pure, natural vitamin E is rather expensive.

3. Vitamin E labeled as "dl" instead of "d" is synthetic and of little value. Man has not yet been able to duplicate natural E.

4. The only type of vitamin E with proven antioxidant activity is natural vitamin E extract. This extract is made primarily from soybean oil. The vitamin E is distilled out of the oil. This extract, if left unaltered, is potent in antioxidant activity. Unfortunately, over 90% of the vitamin E on the market is esterified, i.e. chemically altered. Chemists bind the vitamin E molecule to substances known as acetate or succinate. Through this method, the shelf life is greatly increased while the antioxidant activity is diminished.

5. Read all labels. Select only those products listing their vitamin E as being non-esterified. These unaltered vitamin E products are known as free tocopherols, mixed tocopherols, alpha tocopherol, etc.*

SCIENTIFIC STUDIES PROVE
THE WORTH OF ANTIOXIDANTS

There are literally thousands of scientific articles written by medical and nutritional researchers documenting various beneficial effects which antioxidants have on health. Every week, hundreds more of these articles are published. Antioxidants as a primary treatment and cure for degenerative disease is the wave of the future. Let me quote some examples from this wealth of scientific data.

1. The researchers Kikuchi and Koyama found that high fat diets in rabbits caused the rabbits' red blood cells to become deformed due to free radical damage. However, when the rabbits were given vitamin E, the red blood cells stayed normal, even though the high fat diet was continued. Vitamin E, therefore, acted as an antioxidant, protecting the red blood cell membrane from being damaged.

2. Drs. Manwaring and Csallany showed that organs which receive lots of oxygen such as the brain, lungs, and liver are damaged by the oxygen *if the organs are deficient in vitamin E.* The addition of vitamin E protected the organs from this damage. Apparently, the liver was most sensitive to the oxygen-induced damage. This may be one reason why the liver serves as the main depot for vitamin E storage.

3. Researchers Whitacre and Combs found that a deficiency of selenium leads to pancreatic damage. The actual outer membranes of the pancreatic cells become destroyed due to the ill effects of free radicals, which are toxic to the cell membranes. Damage to the

* A few brands are available which contain only free tocopherols (see appendix B).

pancreas is critical, as no food can be properly digested without it. You may recall that in every cell in your body, there is an enzyme which protects cell membranes from free radical damage — glutathione peroxidase. Selenium is needed for this enzyme to work properly, and its deficiency greatly diminishes glutathione peroxidase activity. In severe selenium deficiency, the internal organs are left literally unprotected. In most instances, supplementation with selenium rapidly reverses the damage.

4. Sickle cell anemia is caused, in part, by free radical-induced damage to the cell walls of red blood cells. Rachmitewitz and his colleagues proved that vitamin E at 400 I.U. per day resulted in a decrease in the number of sickled cells in patients with this disease. Apparently, vitamin E acts to prevent healthy red blood cells from turning into sickle cells. This is truly amazing since sickle cell anemia has been regarded for years by the medical profession as being incurable.

5. The Journal of the American Medical Association reported recently that vitamin E supplements are effective in fibrocystic disease of the breasts. The breasts are vulnerable to free radical damage, since free radicals love to attack polyunsaturated fats and the breasts are primarily made up of fatty tissue. Vitamin E apparently blocks this damage, although it would be more effective if combined with selenium.

6. Dr. Prasad found that the growth of melanoma tumor cells on animals was blocked by vitamin E. He suggested that fat-soluble antioxidants such as beta carotene and vitamin E alter the physics of the cell membrane of cancer cells, leading to an inhibition of their growth.

7. Drs. Collip and Chen showed that selenium deficiency leads to heart damage in both children and adults, and that it is not uncommon for either of these age groups to become selenium deficient. Much of this damage is corrected when selenium levels in the blood and tissues are increased.

8. Researchers Lloyd and Clayton have shown that both smoking and alcohol use lead to a selenium deficiency. It is likely that the selenium is "used up" in an attempt to heal the tissue damage caused by cigarette smoke and/or alcohol.

9. Tiny arteries in the retina of the eye are vulnerable to damage from various noxious agents. Once these arteries are damaged severely, vision is affected, and partial or complete blindness can result. This does occur in diseases such as diabetes and macular degeneration. The researcher Thornber and his colleagues found that a high-sugar diet in animals damages the retinal arteries leading to visual

impairment and blindness. It is known that sugar causes this in humans as well. For example, sugar diabetes is the number one cause of blindness in America today. However, these researchers discovered that selenium protected the animals against damage to the retinal arteries, even though the nurient-poor, sugar-rich diet was continued. They also added chromium which, while not technically an antioxidant, does help prevent sugar-induced damage to the eyes.

10. Dr. Prasad demonstrated that levels of cancer-causing chemicals in the digestive tract are reduced by vitamins C, E, and A.

11. Many researchers have shown that vitamin E decreases the incidence of breast tumors. Vitamin E is soluble in fat and will dissolve into breast tissue, protecting it from free radical-induced damage.

12. Recently, researchers have proven that high levels of beta carotene, folic acid, and B-12 diminish the odds for the development of lung cancer. Deficiencies of B-12 and, particularly, folic acid are common — and you can bet that all smokers and drinkers are deficient. Both of these B-vitamins modify the rate at which cells reproduce, keeping the cells "under control" and helping prevent the onset of cancer.

13. Researchers Griffin and Lane showed that persons working around toxic chemicals known as *hydrocarbons* (oil and coal derivatives) had lower selenium and glutathione peroxidase levels than did the normal population. Both of these are needed by the liver to detoxify hydrocarbons, which are often difficult to remove from the tissues.

14. Numerous researchers have determined that a lack of selenium and, thus, a lack of glutathione peroxidase, leads to skin damage, and may even cause skin diseases. The skin's fatty-acid coat is protected from damage by the sun, radiation, and/or free radicals by selenium, and also vitamin E and beta carotene. Treatment of diseases such as eczema, psoriasis, vasculitis (inflammation of the blood vessels in the skin), and seborrheic dermatitis with selenium and vitamin E leads to a beneficial effect in many cases.

15. Deficiencies of antioxidants lead to damage of the blood vessels, particularly the arteries. This was illustrated in 1980 by Dr. Goto who determined that damage to the inner lining of the arteries, leading to hardening of the arteries and even stroke is often due to excess lipid peroxides circulating in the blood. Lipid peroxides, as described earlier in this chapter, are fats which have become so toxic that they damage the fatty acids of healthy cell membranes throughout the body. These lipid peroxides are rapidly abolished by the addition of prodigious quantities of antioxidants, particularly selenium, vitamin E, vitamin C, and beta carotene to the diet.

16. High vitamin E levels in the blood are associated with protection from heart disease, arterial damage, cataracts, cancer, and pollution-induced cell damage. The blood levels necessary to achieve these protective effects are much higher than could ever result from consuming the RDA (Recommended Daily Allowance). A recent study showed that doses of vitamin E up to 60 times the RDA (1000 I.U.) were required to provide maximum protection from these and other free radical-induced diseases. Need there be any more debate? With our toxic world as it is today, only a fool would believe that he will get by through consuming only the RDA. By the standards described above, the RDA for vitamin E (10-15 I.U.) is worthless.

17. Dr. H. Garewal of the University of Arizona recently showed that supplements of natural beta carotene caused pre-cancerous lesions in the mouth to disappear. When patients stop taking the beta carotene, the lesions recurred.

REMARKABLE FACTS ABOUT ANTIOXIDANTS

The following are some interesting functions which antioxidants perform in the body:

FUNCTION	ANTIOXIDANT
1. Preservation of the elastic nature of skin	selenium, pantothenic acid, vitamin C
2. Increased ability of brain cells to use oxygen	glutathione, vitamine E. coenzyme Q-10
3. Improved ability of cells to make energy	selenium, vitamin E, glutathione, coenzyme Q-10
4. Detoxification of ozone and radiation	beta carotene, selenium, glutathione, SOD.
5. Enhancement of the immune system	beta carotene, selenium, vitamin E, glutathione, vitamin C pantothenic acid
6. Improved blood flow to the heart	vitamin E coenzyme Q-10
7. Prevention of cancer	all antioxidants
8. Dissolving moles and brown spots	selenium, glutathione
9. Destruction of tumor cells	beta carotene, glutathione, selenium

The importance of antioxidants has been made clear. They have hundreds of known and many unknown functions. You can see why it would be wise to add these protective nutrients to your diet. Load up on antioxidant-rich foods and supplements. It may well be the best investment you'll ever make.

CHAPTER 7
The Number One Killer

I do not deny that many advances have been made in the treatment of heart disease. Yet despite it all, cardiovascular disease remains the number one cause of death. There must be a reason.

Other cultures, even some relatively modern ones, do not have such a problem. Could there be a difference in lifestyle among these societies? In fact, the number one difference between our culture and cultures where heart disease is non-existent is diet. To many this may not be much of a surprise. However, let me give some examples for those who find this hard to believe.

The people of Crete, an island in the Mediterranean, have a high-fat diet that is rich in natural, unprocessed foods. They enjoy good health and longevity. They are free of coronary artery disease. The incidence of stroke or high blood pressure is also minimal.

The Masai tribesmen of Africa eat large quantities of beef and drink whole milk regularly. Only when they migrate to Westernized cities do they develop coronary artery disease, high blood pressure, and atherosclerosis.

The Yemeni Jews, despite a diet rich in natural fats including butter, did not develop circulatory diseases until they moved to Israel. The Israeli diet is very similar to the American one.

The Eskimos are entirely free of coronary artery disease, heart attack, stroke, and high blood pressure even though their diet is rich in such things as seal and whale blubber. Those who now live on white bread, sugar, coffee, tea and alcohol are developing all sorts of "modern" diseases.

Several societies in the Mediterranian are free of heart or circulatory disease, though their diet is up to 70% fat. The same is true for certain Eastern European cultures.

In the past 20 years, attempts have been made by medical men and the media to lay the blame on fats in our diet. Fats are only a part of the problem, although for the societies mentioned, they pose no problem at all. What else, then, in our diet is to blame?

SUGAR IS MORE DANGEROUS THAN FAT

While fat can be natural, sugar is dangerous because it is always unnatural. White sugar is a refined food and has no nutritional value. In fact, its consumption actually leads to a removal of nutrients from the body.

Dr. Yudkin, a famous British researcher, has proven that ill effects upon the circulatory system occur from the consumption of white sugar. He has shown that sugar causes all types of heart and arterial disease. These harmful effects result whether the sugar is obvious (a teaspoon of sugar in your tea) or hidden (a doughnut, some ketchup, or a piece of bologna). No doubt, some people are more vulnerable to its ill-effects than others. One way or the other, a heavy intake of sugar will compromise your health.

SUGAR STRESSES THE ADRENAL AND THYROID GLANDS

While you may not develop heart disease, the sugar you eat will wear down other critical organs. Both the adrenal and thyroid glands must deal with the physiological upset that pure sugar causes in the body. Eventually, if sugar consumption does not stop, these delicate organs will burn themselves out. It so happens that most people with heart disease have malfunctioning thyroid and adrenal glands.

SOME FATS ARE BAD

Unfortunately, many of the fats which Americans get in their diets are toxic to the circulatory system. These "bad fats" may be of either animal or vegetable origin. Other societies have the luxury of consuming large amounts of the helpful or "good" fats. But fat, by itself, is not the killer. I will discuss this in more depth in Chapter 12.

THE AMERICAN DIET — A PROMOTER OF HEART DISEASE

Our diet is the number one factor predisposing us to heart disease. There are many elements within the diet that make us more vulnerable.

I have devised a questionnaire that you can use to determine if your lifestyle is predisposing you to cardiovascular disease, a category which includes coronary heart disease, heart attack, stroke and/or high blood pressure.

WHAT ARE YOUR RISKS? THIS TEST WILL TELL.

ANSWER YES OR NO TO THE FOLLOWING QUESTIONS. ADD
UP THE POINTS TO ARRIVE AT YOUR SCORE.

POINTS

Do you eat fatty or deep-fried foods? .... (5)

Do you regularly eat bakery goods such as doughnuts,
cupcakes, pies, cookies, cakes, etc.? .... (5)

Do you eat cured meats such as bacon, hot dogs, bologna,
sausage, ham, or corned beef? .... (5)

Do you regularly consume sugar added to foods, coffee, or tea,
or in cereals, pop, candy, chocolate, etc.? .... (10)

Do you regularly drink alcoholic beverages? .... (10)

Do you smoke cigarettes? .... (10)

Were you previously a smoker or drinker? .... (5)

Do you have a family history of heart disease, high blood
pressure, or stroke? .... (10)

Do you have a family history of elevated blood fats, cholesterol
or triglycerides? .... (10)

Are you considerably overweight (i.e. greater than 20 pounds)? .. (10)

Do you lead a sedentary life (i.e. little or no exercise)? .... (5)

Do you have elevated cholesterol and/or triglycerides? .... (20)

Do you have high blood pressure (above 140/90)? .... (25)

Have you recently had a stroke or heart attack? .... (50)

Are you currently diagnosed as having heart disease, heart
failure, enlarged heart, blood clots, or hardening of
the arteries? .... (50)

Do you have symptoms of poor circulation such as memory loss,
sluggish mental function, chest pain, shortness of breath, cold
extremities, or leg pains/cramps? .... (15)

Do you regularly take birth control pills? .... (10)

Have you used drugs such as water pills, diet pills,
marijuana, cocaine, or heroin for an extended period
in the past or do you currently use them? .... (5)

Do you drink coffee in excess of 5 cups a day? .... (5)

YOUR SCORE

10-35 POINTS   Possible cardiovascular disease. Treatment would be preventive.

40-65 POINTS   Probable cardiovascular disease. Treatment is needed. Failure to alter lifestyle and improve the diet could lead to significant disease. Stop the progression now before it is too late. Proper treatment at this stage could reverse much of the damage.

70-135 POINTS   You have definite evidence of cardiovascular disease. Treatment is mandatory. Your risk for further health complications is high. Failure to alter your lifestyle, diet, and nutrition could be life-threatening.

140-ABOVE DANGER — HIGH RISK!   Stroke, heart attack, hypertensive crisis, or other cardiovascular complications could occur at any time. It is imperative that you alter your lifestyle and seek medical care immediately. However, do not expect the doctors to offer any miracle cure. The burden of cure rests with you. Well-planned changes in your dietary, nutritional, and exercise habits *could save your life!*

You can see from this test that a number of factors play a role in causing heart disease. For twenty years the medical profession and news media have pounded the public on the subject of cholesterol, indicating that its excess in the diet causes heart disease. I will now expose what I call the cholesterol hoax.

CHOLESTEROL IS *NOT* THE CULPRIT

Are my words controversial? Of course. Can I provide proof for what I am saying? Absolutely. Cholesterol in and of itself does not cause heart disease. That's right. Cholesterol is an important substance made by the body. It has a variety of useful functions. Every cell in our bodies contains cholesterol. Without it, our cells would be vulnerable to disease, infection, and even cancer. How could such an important, natural substance be deemed so harmful?

Cholesterol first got its bad rap when it was found that many people with disease, not just heart disease, had high blood cholesterol. From this it was assumed by doctors and nutritionists that cholesterol was bad and that the cure would be, in part, the removal of cholesterol from the diet. This way of thinking is not much different than to assume that when the water level in a river is high, it is bad, and when it is low, it is good. No doubt, there is more danger of a flood if the water level is up, but that does not mean that the water itself is bad! The same is true of cholesterol. While its elevation is an indication of disturbed function and is associated with increased risk of certain diseases (including heart disease), it is likely that it is the *body* that is bad, not the cholesterol.

What I mean is that often the cholesterol is elevated for a reason. Its elevation may be serving a useful function. This is because cholesterol itself is an antioxidant. It is made in the liver according to the body's needs. Too low of a cholesterol level is as dangerous as too high. The proof is in. Extremely low cholesterol is associated with breakdowns in the immune system and cancer. This is brought out best by the fact that drugs which artificially lower cholesterol cause a number of cancers. To reiterate, every cell and organ in the body needs an adequate amount of cholesterol to remain free of disease. The immune cells in particular need a steady supply of this valuable nutrient. If your cholesterol level is too high or low, the following charts may be of interest to you.

CAUSES OF HIGH CHOLESTEROL LEVELS

1. Excess dietary sugar

2. Excess dietary starch

3. Excess hydrogenated or processed fats (lard. shortening. cottonseed oil. palm oil. margarine. etc.)

4. Liver dysfunction

5. Amino acid deficiency

6. Essential fatty acid deficiency

7. Deficiency of natural antioxidants such as vitamin E. selenium. and beta carotene

8. Increased tissue damage due to infection. radiation. or oxidative activity (free radicals, etc.)

9. Fiber deficiency

10. Vitamin C deficiency

11. Carnitine deficiency

12. Biotin deficiency

13. Food allergies

14. Alcoholism

CAUSES OF LOW CHOLESTEROL LEVELS (below 150)

1. Immune decline

2. Chronic hepatitis

3. Cholesterol-lowering drugs

4. Essential fatty acid deficiency

5. Liver infection or disease

6. Manganese deficiency

7. Adrenal stress

8. Street drugs (cocaine. marijuana, etc.)

9. Excessive exercise (especially in females)

10. Low fat diets

11. Psychological stress

12. Cancer*

As you can see, cutting out the eggs is not the answer. If you have a cholesterol problem, a much better step is finding out why imbalances in your chemistry exist. You can also see that causing the cholesterol to drop too low is not wise.

WHERE DOES CHOLESTEROL COME FROM?

Most of the cholesterol found in the blood is made within our own bodies. The liver synthesizes more cholesterol each day than can possibly be absorbed from the diet. The equivalent of ten or more eggs worth per day are manufactured under normal conditions. This cholesterol is used to seal off damaged tissues, arterial walls, and cell membranes. It is also utilized in the synthesis of adrenal hormones. In addition, cholesterol is a vital component of nerve and brain tissue. Most people are not aware that you can actually have a cholesterol deficiency, and that this deficiency can damage the heart! The heart cannot function adequately unless the nerves which control it are healthy — a state dependent on an adequate supply of cholesterol and other nerve-nourishing substances.

HOW DIET INFLUENCES CHOLESTEROL LEVELS

Another source of cholesterol is diet. Do I mean foods high in cholesterol? Not really. Most foods naturally rich in cholesterol such as eggs, fresh meats, liver, and butterfat do not cause a significant increase in blood cholesterol levels. Are you astonished? You shouldn't be, because if you think about it, it makes a lot of sense. At the beginning of this chapter, a number of examples were given of societies whose diets are high in unprocessed fats, and, yet, these societies have low mortality from heart disease. These people also have normal cholesterol levels despite eating a variety of cholesterol-rich foods. There are several reasons for this effect:

* Very low levels of cholesterol, especially below 130 have been associated with increased cancer risk. Cholesterol is needed to protect cells from damage by radiation, toxins, viruses, and other substances which can initiate cancer.

1. Cholesterol-rich foods contain certain natural substances which actually lower blood cholesterol and assist the body in the metabolism of fats. This would include such compounds as lecithin, essential fatty acids, manganese, and carnitine.

2. When cholesterol is eaten, the body recognizes this, and by an amazing mechanism reduces or shuts down cholesterol synthesis in the liver.

3. Most cholesterol-rich foods (butter, eggs, organ meats, shellfish) are rich in a variety of other nutrients. Often, these foods are listed within one of the categories of the wholesome, basic food groups. Eliminating them more often than not means their replacement by less nutritious foods (i.e. Egg-Beater's vs. real eggs)

4. Most of the foreign diets which are high in fat and cholesterol are also low in refined sugars and starches. In contrast, the American diet is high in fats as well as refined sugars and starches. Cholesterol levels increase if the diet is high in either sugars or starches, since the liver makes cholesterol from the breakdown products of sugar.

SUGAR RAISES CHOLESTEROL LEVELS

Now you have it! The truth is, whatever *causes* an abnormal elevation in blood cholesterol is bad. Refined carbohydrates of all types lead to an elevation of blood fats. These include white sugar, brown sugar, malt, corn syrup, corn starch, maltodextrin, dextrose, glucose, white flour, and white rice. Hundreds of case histories and many research studies have proven that these depleted foods cause an elevation in cholesterol and/or triglycerides by a phenomenon I call glucose overload.

HOW DOES SUGAR END UP AS FAT?

All the above-mentioned carbohydrates are broken down by the body into a single common substance — glucose. Starch is nothing more than a chain of glucose molecules. These chains are broken apart by digestive enzymes. Sugar is made up of single molecules (glucose, dextrose, etc.) or double molecules, such as white sugar (sucrose). Sucrose is broken down by digestive enzymes into glucose and fructose. This is where the phenomenon of glucose overload comes in.

When you take in more glucose (or fructose) than you can burn as energy, the body has no choice but to process it into stored energy: fat. This connection is best illustrated by the following case history:

MR. JACOBS, RETIRING EXECUTIVE

Mr. Jacobs came to me for one reason: he was scared to death of undergoing by-pass surgery. There was reason for him to be concerned:

he was constantly plagued with angina pains. Recently, he underwent two coronary angioplasties, operations where the cardiologist tries to open clogged coronary arteries with a plastic catheter. Both of these procedures had failed. He was placed on medications and given the standard heart-saver diet used by hospitals and their dieticians.

I attempted to find out *why* Mr. Jacobs had this problem. Although he never had a heart attack, he was a mild diabetic and was grossly overweight. He was a sugar addict supreme, reveling in all sorts of candies and sweets. Even though he didn't drink or smoke, he did follow a poor diet which was likely the cause of his heart troubles. He was, in every sense of the word, a "sweet heart."

Testing showed that Mr. Jacobs was actually allergic to sugar. Whenever he ate sugar or other refined carbohydrates, his triglycerides sky-rocketed to as high as 1000! Due to his exteme addiction to sugar, Mr. Jacobs was a tough nut to crack. Yet, being a businessman, he was accustomed to discipline. Mr. Jacobs was placed on a diet free of all sugars and starches. Instead, he was instructed to eat foods such as vegetables, meats, and low-sugar fruits. Needless to say, his triglycerides came down to normal in no time. He dropped 25 pounds, his heart pain improved, and he is now able to exercise and take long walks, though prior to his therapy he was relatively debilitated. Had these problems been discovered and addressed earlier, the risky coronary angioplasties could have been avoided. As far as by-pass surgery goes, I do not think Mr. Jacobs would have lived through it. Currently, Mr. Jacobs, having kept to his diet, has lost nearly 50 pounds and is walking over 5 miles a day — without any angina. Needless to say, Mr. Jacobs is indeed happily retired.

TRIGLYCERIDES

For the heart patient, this term is the companion evil to cholesterol. What is a triglyceride? It is a fat formed from three (therefore the "tri") fatty acids attached to a molecule known as glycerol. Most of the triglycerides found in the body do not come directly from dietary fats per se; they are made in the liver from any excess sugar which hasn't been burned. As has been stated, glucose and many other sugars originate from processed foods. These sugars can also come from whole foods which naturally contain carbohydrates. This includes the natural sugars in milk, the starch of a baked potato, or the sugar in a bunch of grapes. In a vulnerable person, any of these foods could lead to elevated triglycerides.

Most Americans get an excess of starch and/or sugar in their diets. Unless you are a marathon athlete or a college wrestler, it is likely that you are not burning up the sugar you eat fast enough. The extra sugar will enter the liver and will then be synthesized into fat. While this extra fat may not be a critical thing for a healthy person, it is deadly to the individual afflicted with heart disease.

These extra fats may not make it to the front of your abdomen or the outside of your hips. Unfortunately, they are often deposited in organs of crucial function: the liver, arteries, brain, and heart.

The liver is the factory responsible for making important molecules known as *carrier proteins*. These proteins are responsible for carrying minerals, vitamins, and fatty acids, such as cholesterol or triglycerides in the blood. The well known HDL ("good") and LDL ("bad") cholesterol are carrier proteins made in the liver. A malfunctioning liver cannot make sufficient quantities of HDL cholesterol, and a liver infiltrated with fat is not able to work up to speed. The less HDL cholesterol you have, the more likely it is that fats will be deposited into your arteries.

In the worst scenario, fats plug up the arteries in the heart, leading to angina, sudden death, or heart attack. However, more likely causes of heart problems would be as follows:

HEART DISEASE IS OFTEN A BIOCHEMICAL DISORDER

Dr. Cooley, the noted cardiovascular surgeon from Texas stated that no more than 20% of all heart attacks are due to occluded coronary arteries. Thus, blood clots and fat deposits play only a partial role. What, then, accounts for the other 80%? Likely causes are biochemical and nutritional imbalances within the heart itself, or in organs which support cardiac functions. Medical men have long associated disorders of the thyroid gland with heart disease. Emotional and psychic stress, with its powerful effects upon the brain and nervous system play a major role as well.

The health of the liver has a great bearing upon diseases of circulation. As stated previously, the liver synthesizes HDL and LDL cholesterol. These are also known as lipoproteins since they are made from protein and fats, i.e., lipids. Much of the fatty acid metabolism in the body is controlled by the liver. It synthesizes carnitine and taurine, nutrients critical of importance to the heart.

CARNITINE — FAT BURNER

For years, people seeking to lose weight effortlessly have searched for a miracle pill to burn off excess fat. Little did they know that nature makes its own fat burner — carnitine. Carnitine is an amino acid made primarily in the liver. It is used to carry fats into cells, so they can be used for their primary purpose — as a source of fuel. Fats cannot be properly combusted without adequate amounts of carnitine.

HEARTS LOVE FAT

You may have a lovely heart, but did you know that your heart loves fat? The primary fuel used by the heart is fat. It specializes in the oxidation of fats into energy. Few people are aware of this fact, although it has been known by medical science for decades. No one is sure why the heart prefers fats above all other fuels. Possibly fats are a more efficient form of energy. The heart needs to be efficient in its energy production more so than any other organ. After all, our hearts never sleep — if your heart stopped to take a breather, you would be dead! The heart pumps 13,000 pints of fluid throughout the body each day. With this huge workload, it needs to have the most effective energy conservation mechanism possible. Fats *are* the most productive source, providing over twice the amount of energy per gram as do sugars, starches, or proteins. Here again, the health of your heart depends upon a properly functioning liver — enter carnitine. Carnitine binds to the fatty acids and carries them into the heart's muscle cells. Once reaching the mitochondria, tiny factory-like organs located within the cells, carnitine releases the fatty acids. The mitochondria which are found within the heart cells in great numbers then burn the fats into energy. This energy is used to keep the heart pumping. Remember, the heart is the only organ in the body that *never gets to rest.*

Those who promote a low fat, high-carbohydrate diet for heart disease never take the above mentioned facts into account. They neglect a most fundamental part of normal human physiology — that heart tissue prefers to utilize fat above all other dietary sources of caloric energy. Foods rich in fats such as meats, chicken, eggs, and nuts contain carnitine and other nutrients which help the body metabolize the fats which they naturally contain. This is another principle that the anti-natural fat dieticians and nutritionists fail to grasp.

Carnitine is made in the liver from two amino acids; lysine and methionine. These amino acids are in the category known as "essential" amino acids. This means that the body cannot make them. Thus, you must get them in the diet. Without sufficient lysine or methionine, a carnitine deficiency will result. Vitamin C is also needed for the carnitine synthesis reaction to proceed.

SUGAR: THE POOR MAN'S FUEL

From this you can see that the heart is dependent upon fats, proteins (amino acids), and vitamins and does not need even a pinch of sugar. Sugar damages the heart in the following ways:

1. It depletes valuable minerals from the body, minerals helpful to cardiac function.

2. It takes up calories in the diet where heart-nourishing calories are needed.

3. It disrupts protein metabolism and interferes with carnitine synthesis.

4. It destroys B-vitamins needed by the heart, such as thiamine, biotin, pyridoxine, and niacin.

5. It leads to the production of excess quantities of triglycerides and other fats which could end up being deposited in the arteries.

6. Its use can lead to the development of high blood pressure which places added stress on the heart.

7. It causes hardening of the arteries which doubles or even triples the energy it takes for the heart to pump blood through the arterial system.

DIETARY SOURCES OF CARNITINE

The consequences of carnitine deficiency are many. In essence, fats can pile up throughout the arteries and within the cells, since without this key nutrient, they cannot be fully metabolized. The liver does make some carnitine on a daily basis. Vegetarians with high cholesterol and triglycerides are likely carnitine deficient, since few vegetables contain more than a trace of it. Meat products constitute the major sources. Here is a comprehensive listing of carnitine-rich foods:

ANIMAL PRODUCTS	**PLANT SOURCES**
Lamb meat and fat	Avocado
(the richest known source)	(the richest vegetable source)
Beef	Brewer's yeast
Liver, heart and other organ meats	Wheat germ
Whole milk	Peanuts
Cream chicken or turkey breast	Cauliflower
Fish	Cabbage

In addition, carnitine supplements may be useful. Research has shown that supplemental carnitine is particularly valuable for lowering triglyceride levels. Other conditions responding favorably include mitral valve prolapse, high blood pressure, heart failure, and coronary artery disease. Some cases of cardiac arrhythmia also respond to carnitine supplementation. Carnitine can also help raise HDL cholesterol levels, while lowering total cholesterol.

Carnitine-rich foods should be added freely to the diet despite their obvious fat content. Losses of carnitine from food due to cooking can be considerable. Meat, if cooked excessively, loses most of its carnitine. Broiled meats lose their carnitine in the juices; do pour the juices from the bottom of the pan over your meats. Make gravies with these juices and do not throw them out for fear of their fat content.*

*I don't recommend adding white flour to your gravies. Try adding rice bran instead or use whole wheat flour.

Avocado is a great source of carnitine since it is usually eaten uncooked. What little carnitine is found in cauliflower and cabbage is lost in cooking unless they are steamed or eaten raw.

LAMB FAT — A NEW HEART SAVER?

Eat your lamb chops nice and juicy and don't trim off any of the fat: that lamb fat is just loaded with carnitine. For centuries people in Palestine and Greece made use of every part of their lambs, fat included. They rendered this fat and kept it to be used for cooking. Heart disease was nonexistent despite their eating pure fat!

Of course, I don't recommend that you start eating pure animal fat of any kind. But I do suggest that you eat your fill of lamb without trimming the visible fat! It tastes better that way. Try to eat your lamb chops and steaks medium-rare. Remember, well done meat loses much of its carnitine.

LARD: THE HEART'S DOOM

Lard is bad for the heart. It is a processed fat and is added relatively freely to our food supply. Many deep-frying fats contain lard. Whenever you see the word "shortening" on a label, you can bet it contains lard. Lard is harmful in part because it easily becomes rancid. It also contains a high fraction of polyunsaturated fats which are quite toxic.

Lard has no nutritional value. It would be best to keep it on the pig and out of the human body.

PROTEIN IS GOOD FOR THE HEART

If you are plagued with heart disease, high blood pressure, or hardening of the arteries, you probably need more protein. Is this contrary to popular opinion? Yes! We have been told that we get too much protein. To a degree this may be true. But I believe we are not getting enough high quality protein. Let me explain.

If 40 to 80% of the diet is in the form of deep fried fat, greasy foods, chips, snacks, flour, sugar, and sweets, then something has to give. These foods have to replace something. That something usually is high quality foods such as proteins, vegetables, nuts, and fruits.

How often do you make these high quality proteins a regular part of the diet?

- fish, fresh or frozen
- eggs, whole milk, or cheese (i.e. hard or cottage)
- fermented whole milk products
- chicken (baked or broiled)
- beef or lamb
- bee pollen, sunflower seeds, or pumpkin seeds
  fresh nut meats and nut butters

If you are losing portions of these excellent protein foods, you may have become deficient in certain components of proteins needed to maintain cardiovascular fitness. I have mentioned carnitine. The amino acids it is made from (lysine and methionine) are found primarily in high-quality protein foods such as those listed on the previous page.

Animal proteins are the primary source for both of these amino acids, especially methionine. A few plants are rich in lysine, including soybeans, oatmeal, and lentils.

TAURINE: ANOTHER UNIQUE AMINO ACID

Taurine is another important nutrient derived from proteins. Like carnitine, it is synthesized by the liver. However, in contrast to carnitine, dietary sources of taurine are inadequate for supplying worthwhile amounts. We have to depend almost entirely on the liver's ability to synthesize it from another amino acid: cysteine. Fortunately, cysteine is found in a wide variety of foods, particularly animal proteins.

The heart and blood vessels need taurine. Just as carnitine carries fats, taurine carries minerals into the cells. Minerals can be lost from the body in many ways. Sugar, for example, causes the loss of potassium and magnesium in the urine. Taurine helps prevent the loss of these valuable, life-saving minerals by binding them tightly within the cells.

SUDDEN DEATH AND TAURINE DEFICIENCY

This is a story you have probably heard of before. An aspiring executive of a major corporation dies of sudden cardiac standstill, leaving behind his wife and children. Was it preventable? I say yes, and taurine may well be a major player in this scene. Patients admitted to the hospital with acute chest pains had significantly higher concentrations of taurine in their blood than did normal people. You are probably wondering how a taurine deficiency could be represented by an increase in blood levels. It is because taurine is deficient within the cells. When the body is under stress, taurine is lost from the cells into the bloodstream and eventually is excreted into the urine. Most cases of sudden death or heart attack occur during stressful events. Once taurine is depleted, valuable minerals such as calcium, potassium, and magnesium are easily washed out of cells. Without these minerals, the nerves of the heart become irritable and unstable. Thus, a fatal cardiac arrhythmia can result. Do you remember the deaths that occurred when dieters were using the liquid protein diet? Many of the fatalities were due to cardiac arrhythmia, which resulted in sudden death. These formulas were composed of incomplete proteins and contain no taurine. It is likely that the lack of taurine led to potassium deficiency, and that this was the actual cause for these unfortunate deaths.

MEDICAL USES FOR TAURINE

Taurine keeps the nerve and muscle cells of the heart calm. It helps the cells of the body hold onto the minerals they so desperately need. No surprise, then, that taurine has been found useful in the treatment of a variety of diseases including:

1. High blood pressure
2. Congestive heart failure
3. Heart rhythm disturbances
4. Atherosclerosis
5. Epilepsy
6. Gallbladder disease
7. Alzheimer's disease

SOURCES OF TAURINE

Goat's and cow's milk contain some taurine. However, the only significant source is in mother's milk which contains ten times that found in cow's milk. It is likely that, with the recent baby-boomer explosion, statistics will show in 20 to 30 years that breast-fed babies will have a far less incidence of heart disease or high blood pressure than those fed formula or cow's milk.

Many excellent taurine supplements are available in the marketplace. I have listed the companies I recommend in appendix B. In addition, I advise all cardiac patients to take a daily dose of vitamins B-2 and B-6, since the liver needs them to synthesize taurine. In addition, vitamin B-12, magnesium, and zinc are needed for taurine to be properly metabolized. Last but not least, make sure you consume enough high quality protein foods.

WATCH OUT FOR THE MINERAL THIEVES

Simple sugars and refined starches, such as white flour and rice, cause the loss of cardio-protective minerals, while high-quality foods such as proteins, fruits, and vegetables help you retain them. A list of substances which steal heart-nourishing minerals out of the body includes:

- white sugar
- corn syrup
- white flour
- distilled water
- coffee
- ice tea
- soft drinks
- some forms of fiber (if taken in excess)
- diuretics

DIURETICS MAY WASH YOUR LIFE AWAY

Are you taking water pills for your heart trouble? Water pills, known by the medical term *diuretics*, can be very dangerous. Many fatalities in the elderly are due to the side-effects of these drugs. The reason they are so dangerous is that they wash out valuable nutrients such as potassium, magnesium, and sodium. If tissue levels of any of these minerals become too low, sudden death or stroke can occur.

Nature has provided many diuretics which can remove excess fluid without adverse effects. Taurine was mentioned as a useful treatment for congestive heart failure, a condition where fluids overload the heart and lungs. Potassium itself has a diuretic action, as does magnesium. Many herbs stimulate the kidneys to eliminate water. A partial list includes alfalfa, uva ursi, parsley, and strawberry leaves. Watermelon is an excellent diuretic, and chlorophyll, which is found in dark green leafy vegetables, has a gentle but effective stimulating action on the kidneys.

HEART MEDICATIONS AND THE SYMPTOMS THEY CREATE

No reasonable cardiologist or internist will tell you that medicines cure heart disease. At most, medications help relieve some of the symptoms. There are several types of heart medicines, the major categories being beta blockers, calcium-channel blockers, anti-arrhythmics, digitalis compounds, vasodialators, anti-clotting agents, and diuretics. Few doctors have the time to tell you about the side effects these medicines create. The following is a list of the more common symptoms and toxicities caused by their use:

SYMPTOMS
1. indigestion
2. dizziness
3. fatigue
4. headache
5. impotence
6. depression
7. palpitations
8. constipation or diarrhea
9. numbness or pain in the nerves
10. breathing difficulty
11. hair loss

TOXICITIES
1. bone marrow damage
2. blockage of the nerves in the heart
3. liver damage or inflammation
4. kidney damage
5. sudden death (from cardiac arrhythmia)

Did you notice that one of the more common toxic effects of heart medicines is to cause damage to the very organ they are being used to treat? Don't be surprised. Fatal heart attacks have been caused by medicines.

CAUSES OF HEART DISEASE

The factors predisposing individuals to heart attack, heart failure, stroke, and high blood pressure are many, some of which have already been discussed. I would like to review with you these factors in more detail.

I. FAT AND SUGAR INTAKE

The theory that fats in the diet are the primary factor in causing heart disease is just that. This idea was started by a resercher named Ancel Keys. In 1953 he noted that certain cultures whose diets were high in fat also had a high incidence of heart disease. From then on, his theory became accepted as fact. No doubt, there is some truth to the theory, but only on this basis — Americans and other people who have lots of heart disease eat massive quantities of REFINED FATS! That's right. It is not the fat itself, but how it is processed or refined that makes it damaging. That brings us back to the topic of sugar. It is proven that sugar intake is related to the increased incidence of all types of circulatory diseases.

Dr. Yudkin, a former professor of Nutrition and Dietetics at Queen Elizabeth College of London University and now Emeritus Dean of Nutrition, first noticed that many of the same countries who had a high intake of fat had a higher intake of sugar! When looking at fat alone, Yudkin found no evidence that people who had high intakes of saturated fats from foods naturally high in fats such as milk, cheese, eggs, or meat had any greater incidence of heart disease than those who did not eat these foods. What he did find, however, was that high intakes of sugar had a clear-cut relationship to the occurrence of heart disease. Here are the glaring statistics:

DEATHS FROM HEART ATTACKS OR HEART DISEASE PER 100,000 PEOPLE*

Per capita sugar consumption	Deaths
20 lbs. of sugar per year	60 deaths
120 lbs. of sugar per year	300 deaths
150 lbs. of sugar per year	750 deaths

Note the dramatic increase in fatalities as sugar intake increases. The most vulnerable group appears to be men, aged 40 to 65, whose sugar intake is high. Apparently, the younger individuals can withstand the extra sugar, and the older ones have survived despite their sugar intake. Thus, if the sugar is going to get you, it could hit at the prime of your life.

* Currently, the average annual consumption of sugar in the U.S.A. is 130 pounds per person (includes adults and children). This means there are some people consuming in excess of 200 pounds of sugar per year —the equivalent of over 1/2 pound of sugar per day.

You might ask, "Is taking the sugar bowl away the answer?" It is, in part, but hidden sugar is even more of a culprit. Most of the per capita consumption comes from sugar which is blended into the food supply. There are, of course, more obvious sources of hidden sugar, such as a candy bar or a can of pop. So many foods in the supermarket contain sugar that it would take a book twice this size to list them. There is an easier way — just look at the label. If it contains any of these sugar or starch-derivatives, don't buy it:

SUGARS

cane sugar
corn syrup
dextrose
fructose
glucose
levulose
maple syrup
molasses
sucrose
sugar

STARCH ADDITIVES

barley malt
malt syrup
corn starch
dextrin
maltodextrin

Are refined sugars and starches really the villain, you ask? Yes, but they are not the only ones.

II. IRON, IRON, EVERYWHERE

The food processors probably believe they are doing us a favor by "fortifying" our food. After destroying up to 95% of all the nutrients in the foods they refine, they fortify them with only a few of the ones that were originally removed. One of these few is iron. Why are foods such as white flour and rice, cereals as well as various other grain products, fortified with iron? These foods do contain small quantities of naturally-bound iron, though much of it is lost during their refinement. Maybe the foods processors are themselves aghast at the devastation they wreak on the foodstuffs and feel they must do something "in return." Cost-effectiveness is the more likely motive. Thus, they fortify the food with iron in the form of iron sulfate (a by-product of industry and manufacturing) and add a few B-vitamins. While no complaint can be registered against the B-vitamins, the added iron may pose a problem: there is a proven increased risk for heart disease and cancer when there is excess iron within the body.

IRON OVERLOAD: ITS EFFECTS UPON VITAMIN E

Iron is found naturally in water and soil. Certain foods are rich in iron, but they are rich in natural iron. Natural iron exists in a chemical form that is harmless to the body. However, the iron added to food is no different than that found in iron filings — and it is in a chemical form that can cause toxicity. We can see how this works in nature versus how it works with iron additives by the following example. Foods naturally rich in iron often contain significant amounts of vitamin E. This natural iron does no harm to the molecules of vitamin E. However, the iron used in food fortification destroys vitamin E, both in the food to which it is added and within the body. Here again, man is not able to duplicate nature. Natural processes within iron-rich plants such as spinach render the iron harmless once it is absorbed from the soil. Not so with inorganic iron, which is highly reactive within the body.

VITAMIN E, INORGANIC IRON, AND YOUR HEART

Vitamin E is a key nutrient for maintaining a healthy heart. It helps keep blood vessels open by preventing excessive blood clotting. As an antioxidant, it protects the muscle and nerve cells of the heart from damage due to toxic compounds (such as inorganic iron). Vitamin E improves the pumping power of the heart and keeps it from becoming easily fatigued. Oxygenation of the blood is improved by vitamin E. You can see that, as far as diseases of circulation are concerned, it is imperative that you retain whatever vitamin E you have in your body and not destroy it! Most people don't even get the RDA of vitamin E through their diet. This tiny amount is quickly destroyed by any inorganic iron there might be in the food. Thus, in many, there is little or no vitamin E available in the body to protect against heart and circulatory diseases.

FOODS CONTAINING ADDED IRON

Unfortunately, all foods containing wheat flour also contain added iron. The exception is stone-ground wheat flour or products made there of. This includes:

- breads
- muffins
- pastries
- cake mixes
- cookies
- pies
- doughnuts
- malted milk
- pudding
- pasta
- crackers
- noodles
- pancake mixes
- creamed soups
- frozen dinners
- gravies
- pretzels

In addition, most breakfast cereals are fortified with iron. This includes nearly all cereals made with wheat, rice, corn, or barley. Cereals that are not fortified include Shredded Wheat, oatmeal, and some granolas.

If you are eating large amounts of any of theses foods, the added iron is probably destroying most of the vitamin E in your body. Extra doses of vitamin E are needed.

In addition, iron in excess of that needed will be stored and deposited within the body. It can end up in the liver, heart, bloodstream, red and white cells, and even in the skin. Once within the tissues it interacts with harmful compounds called free radicals to cause tissue damage. Apparently, the heart is particularly vulnerable to the ill-effects of iron excess.

No doubt some iron is necessary, particularly for menstruating females. In fact, blood loss is the only way nature can reduce iron stores in the body. This is why excess iron is so dangerous to men. Whatever extra iron they get through the diet (or from vitamins containing iron) ends up building up within the body. This extra iron is thought to be the major reason why women who menstruate do not have near the incidence of heart disease as do men of the same age. This is further proven by the fact that after menopause, women become susceptible to cardiovascular disease. Women who use birth control pills are also at risk. Since menstruation is significantly reduced, their iron stores increase and so do their risks for heart attack, high blood pressure, and stroke.

The best way to tell if you have iron overload is to have a blood test which measures levels of a compound known as *ferritin*. Ferritin is a storage form of iron found circulating in the bloodstream. It is made up of iron bound to protein molecules. Most medical laboratories can measure for it. Levels above 90 mean there is too much iron stored in the body. Remember, if blood levels are high, the tissues themselves are overloaded. Red blood cells use iron in the synthesis of hemoglobin. Once that has been achieved, the excess iron is dumped into areas where it is not needed. It can then act as a catalyst for free radical reactions which are dangerous to the cells and their membranes. It is thought that these reactions eventually damage the cells of the heart and arteries, leading to cardiovascular disease.

If you are not anemic, or if you have a proven case of iron overload (verified by a high ferritin level), it is a good idea to avoid the following:

- white flour fortified with iron
- foods containing white flour
- multiple vitamins with iron
- excess quantities of red meat
- foods containing blood (e.g. blood sausage)
- white rice fortified with iron
- cereals fortified with iron

In addition, I recommend that you get rid of some blood. I don't care how you do it — whether you give it to the blood bank, or have your doctor throw it away. If you have too much iron and you are a male or post-menopausal female, blood-letting is the safest way to go. Is this an old wive's tale re-enacted? Not really. I have listed at the back of this book several scientific articles which provide proof for what I say.

HOW OFTEN SHOULD I HAVE MY BLOOD REMOVED?

That depends on how much extra iron you have in your body. The removal of one pint every six months would do for most, although it may be necessary to draw it as often as once per month. All this, of course, must be done under a doctor's care.

Once the excess iron has been removed, you will enjoy better health. This is because with less iron in the body, there will be a significant reduction in the number of free radical reactions. Minimizing the number of these reactions is important. If free radicals get into the cell nucleus and are allowed to reproduce unchecked, they can damage the genetic material. If the genes or chromosomes are damaged, all sorts of serious problems can result ranging from mutations to cancer.

III. THYROID DISORDERS

Both hypo (too little) and hyper (too much) thyroidism can lead to circulatory diseases. Hardening of the arteries and high blood pressure are commonly related to hypothyroidism, while cardiac arrhythmia is often caused by hyperthyroidism. A fatal type of cardiac arrhythmia can also occur in severe cases of hypothyroidism. This is due to an extreme deficiency of potassium within the nerve cells of the heart. In these cases the hypothyroid condition, if left untreated, leads to a gradual loss of the body's potassium stores.

In hypothyroidism there is often an elevation of cholesterol and triglycerides. This is due to a decreased rate at which food is metabolized. Thus, many hypothyroid patients are overweight. The combination of obesity plus hypothyroidism significantly increases risks for the development of cardiovascular diseases.

Certain foods contain chemicals which block the production of thyroid hormone, particularly raw soybeans, cabbage, broccoli, rutabaga, cauliflower, kale, Brussels sprouts, watercress, and peanuts. Cooking partially inactivates the interfering chemical, known medically as a *goitrogen*. Thus, in most instances it is wise to eat these foods cooked. Raw peanuts or soybeans should never be eaten. Fortunately, peanut butter and soybean products are heated to a high enough degree that the goitrogens are destroyed. If you eat these foods frequently, it is a good idea to supplement the diet with extra iodine, since goitrogens work by blocking iodine absorption by the thyroid gland.

IV. ALCOHOL CONSUMPTION

Alcohol causes heart disease. It directly damages the arterial walls, causing hardening of the arteries as well as causing trauma to the heart muscle itself. Alcohol disrupts liver function and often causes permanent liver damage. A properly functioning liver is absolutely essential for the maintenance of a healthy cardiovascular system. Alcohol also causes direct damage to the heart and causes a disease of its own — alcoholic cardiomyopathy.

It is interesting to note that over the last several years, certain scientific researchers have published data claiming that alcohol has a positive benefit on cardiac function. They base these claims on the fact that alcohol causes a rise in HDL-cholesterol. The researchers have gone so far as to presume that a drink or two of alcohol per day could prevent heart disease and extend the life span. However, these researchers do not take into account that certain people who consume alcohol develop a condition in which the heart muscle degenerates. This is known by the term *cardiomyopathy*. Alcohol depletes thiamine and other B-vitamins from within heart tissue. If levels of thiamine within the nerves of the heart become too low, the muscle fibers which are nourished by the nerves begin to degenerate. Cardiomyopathy has been successfully treated with a nutrient known as coenzyme Q-10. Treatment with selenium has also been shown to help. Thiamine may also be effective. Abstinence from all alcoholic beverages is a must.

If you have high blood pressure and you drink one or more alcoholic beverages per day, guess what? The alcohol is probably causing your blood pressure elevation. The cure is abstinence, combined with dietary changes and nutritional supplements (see Chapter 11).

V. CIGARETTE SMOKING

Most everyone is aware that cigarettes are bad for you. Smoking chokes the supply of oxygen to the lungs, blood, and heart. Less well known is the fact that cigarette smoke destroys vitamins C, E, folic acid, and vitamin A, which are key nutrients for maintaining healthy circulation. In addition, smoking generates harmful free radicals. Your risk for getting a heart attack is far greater if you smoke — you know it and even your insurance company knows it!

WHAT CAN I EAT?

By now, many of you are probably thinking that I have taken away all the "good things" of life, right? Wrong! I have only steered you away from the harmful ones. You can eat, snack, and indulge until you are full — providing you eat foods that are good for you. Now that your mouth is watering, here is a list of some healthy snacks. In addition, I have provided numerous recipes plus Two Weeks of Eating Right in the latter portions of this book.

SNACKS FOR THE CARDIOVASCULAR PATIENT

The following snacks are high in vitamins. minerals. and fiber. There is no need to snack on foods containing added sugars. starches. chemicals. and toxic oils. Notice the emphasis on fresh vegetables. They are the ideal snack for the cardiovascular patient.

Sliced Vegetables

carrots	green peppers	zucchini
celery	red peppers	radishes
cucumbers	pickles	turnips

Sliced Meats

| roast beef | chicken |
| roast lamb | turkey |

Fruits

cantaloupe	honeydew
grapefruit	strawberries
watermelon	papaya
kiwi	guava

Nuts and Seeds

almonds	pecans	pumpkin seeds
Brazil nuts	pine nuts	sunflower seeds
filberts	pistachios	walnuts

OTHER

boiled or poached eggs (preferably farm-fresh)
feta cheese
farmer's or Swiss cheese (contains no dyes)
herring (unsweetened)
olives
sardines
shrimp

NUTRITIONAL SUPPLEMENTS
FOR THE HEART DISEASE PATIENT

FISH OILS — TOO GOOD TO BE TRUE?

The proof is in. Eating two or more servings of fish per week decreases the risk of developing heart disease. Eating fish regularly is a good idea. However. if you really want to decrease your risks. I advise that you take supplemental fish oil. The reason why is that reputable medical journals all over the world are reporting that fish oil supplements protect the heart, decrease blood fats, diminish blood clots, and improve circulation.

Probably the most important benefit that the heart patient can receive from taking fish oils is decreased risk of sudden death due to blood clots. Fish oils, in the proper dosage, will actually act as a blood thinner. Drugs such as aspirin, Heparin, and Coumadin also thin the blood, but they are far more dangerous. Fish oils, if taken properly, are entirely safe. They are nature's blood thinners par excellence!

Only the highest-quality fish oil products should be used. Many poor-grade fish oils are now available in the marketplace. I have listed some companies whose products are of the highest quality (see appendix B).

If you are taking fish oils, you must increase your dose of vitamin E. This is because fish oils become rancid easily unless there is plenty of vitamin E around to protect them.

VITAMINS

Most vitamins play an important role in assisting cardiac function. Vitamins A, C, D, E, thiamine, niacin, B-5, and B-6 appear to be most critical. Thiamine deficiency is an established cause of shortness of breath and arrhythmia. A lack of it even predisposes to angina.

Vitamin B-5 (pantothenic acid) is extremely important since it is needed to keep the adrenal glands healthy. Without it, these glands fail to produce sufficient quantities of certain adrenal hormones which keep the heart pumping strong. I recommend that cardiac patients take at least 1 gram of vitamin B-5 daily.

MINERALS

There is hardly a mineral known that doesn't play a role in assisting cardiovascular function. The list includes calcium, magnesium, zinc, silicon, manganese, copper, potassium, and chromium. Cardiac patients should receive healthy doses of all these minerals. Magnesium, chromium, and manganese are particularly important, since cardiac patients are almost always deficient in them. A special role is played by chromium, since without it, blood fats cannot be properly metabolized. A new chromium is now available. A drawback of most chromium supplements including Brewer's yeast is that very little chromium is absorbed into the bloodstream. Tests have shown that this new type of chromium, known as *chromium picolinate* is absorbed better than any other type. Amazing results have thus far been observed in the reduction of blood fat levels and body fat stores with the use of this supplement. Chromium picolinate is available from Klaire Laboratories or by mail order:

CHROMIUM PICOLINATE
c/o Benbow Fitness
501 Lexington Ave.
Fox River Grove, IL 60021
Ph: (708) 639-3299

RADISHES, NUTS, AND MUSHROOMS
FOR A HEALTHY HEART

What do these foods have in common that is of value to the cardiac patient? They are all rich sources of the mineral selenium. Selenium helps prevent damage to the heart's muscle. Without it, muscles throughout the body tend to degenerate. The heart, being a muscle, is no exception.

Recently, scientists in the Netherlands discovered that heart attack patients, when compared to controls, were found to have significantly lower selenium levels. What's more, these levels were low for up to a year prior to the heart attack.

Selenium probably exerts its protective effects through preventing damage to the heart from those nasty free-radicals (see Chapter 6). Other selenium-rich foods are listed in appendix A in Part III of this book.

CONCLUSION

Many factors in our environment predispose us to a high incidence of the number one killer. Nutritional deficiencies, sugar, fats and oils, alcohol, cigarette smoking, caffeine, heavy metals, and toxic chemicals all play a role. It is wise to avoid as many of these as possible in your quest for preventive cardiovascular health.

CHAPTER 8
The Number Two Killer

C ancer prevention is in. With one out of three Americans getting cancer at some point during their lifetime, the reasons are obvious. Once cancer sets in, it is difficult to eradicate. The only logical solution is to prevent it from occurring at all.

There are many reasons why cancer is so prevalent today. Here are some of the more critical ones.

A HEALTHY DIGESTIVE TRACT:
THE IMPORTANCE OF FIBER

There has been a dramatic decrease in the amount of fiber in the diet over the last century. Low fiber diets are clearly associated with an increased risk of digestive cancers, especially colon and rectal cancer. Breast cancer is much more common in women who have a history of constipation due to low fiber diets. Fiber greatly enhances colonic function and decreases the time that stool and wastes remain in the body. With low fiber diets, fecal matter resides in the colon for extended periods. Normally, food should be digested and its residues eliminated within 24 to 36 hours. However, low fiber diets may result in wastes staying within the intestines for days or even weeks! It is only logical that waste products remaining in the body for that long will lead to tissue damage. The colon and rectum usually bear the brunt of this damage, though more distant organs such as the liver, breasts, or skin are often affected. It has been discovered that wastes can leak from the bowel into the bloodstream. These wastes can then contaminate any organ or tissue in the body.

Decreasing intestinal transit time (the time it takes for food to be digested and eliminated) will result in an improvement in health and will also diminish the chances of getting cancer. The risks for all varieties of cancer are reduced. This is because the health of the immune system is dependent to a great degree upon the ability of the body to remove wastes. The immune system itself has several direct connections to the small intestine and colon. Both of these digestive organs are lined with untold millions of white blood cells. In addition, the intestines contain many immune organs, such as the appendix, which serve a protective function.

The intestines love fiber. Fiber massages the intestinal walls, improving muscle tone and increasing local circulation. Fiber maximizes the removal of poisons and intestinal wastes. It is better to have too much fiber than too little. Some fibers are more gentle on the body than others, but no matter what condition you might have, increase your intake of roughage and fiber. Your life may depend upon it!

THE ROLE OF FRIENDLY BACTERIA

Although fiber is a major factor for intestinal health, it is not the only one. A healthy amount of helpful intestinal microbes are necessary for the colon to function optimally. In fact, most of the weight of each bowel movement is made up of bacteria and other microbes. There are more bacteria in the intestines than there are cells in the body! This underscores the importance of intestinal microbes such as lactobacillus acidophilus and bifidus. These bacteria are beneficial since they perform several useful functions. They aid digestion, synthesize vitamins, decompose carcinogens, and add to the bulk of the stool. If the numbers of these bacteria drop too low, they may be overtaken by potentially harmful ones. Antibiotics are the number one factor causing a decline in the quantity of useful intestinal bacteria. Since most people either take antibiotics medicinally or get them via the food chain, I recommend taking a lactobacillus supplement.* Other valuable sources of these organisms include sauerkraut and fermented milk products.

YOUR THOUGHTS CAN AFFECT YOUR DIGESTION

It is important to have a healthy mental outlook. Digestive and intestinal disorders can have much of their origin in our minds. Stress has a profound effect upon the activity of the digestive glands. Anger, grief, depression, and worry disrupt digestion and, thus, alter body chemistry.

* Red meats, chicken, turkey, and fish are all treated with antibiotics.

Certain chemicals can be released from the brain which have a direct effect on the muscular and skin cells lining the intestinal walls. These substances cause an irritation which leads to nausea, stomach pain, indigestion, and colitis. Negative thoughts, if maintained long enough, increase the susceptibility to cancer. Peace of mind is a prerequisite for digestion and health to be at its best.

TOP SOURCES OF FIBER

There are many sources of fiber that can be used to supplement the diet. It is best to get fiber from food itself. Try to eat a supply of fresh vegetables and fruits daily. There is no better way to get fiber than to eat a fresh, raw carrot or a piece of fiber-rich fruit such as watermelon, strawberries, or apples. Fiber supplements of exceptional value include:

- alfalfa (leaves and seeds)
- chlorella
- ground flax seed
- kelp
- oat bran
- psyllium husks
- rice bran
- wheat bran (assuming you are not allergic to wheat)

Whenever fiber intake increases, so increases the need for fluids. It is recommended that anyone who takes a fiber supplement must drink at least six 10 oz. glasses of water per day. This would be in addition to any other drinks taken, such as warm drinks, milk, juice, etc. Otherwise, you could get more bound up than you were in the first place. Fiber is activated by water. Use the two as a team for the best effect.

DISEASES CAUSED BY A LACK OF FIBER

Since the advent of food processing, that is the use of manufacturing procedures which remove certain nutritional substances from whole foods, there has been a rise in the incidence of degenerative diseases. In Chapter 2, the negative effect food processing has on vitamin/mineral content was discussed. Yet fiber is also a nutrient, and food processing removes most of it. The following is a list of diseases resulting from low-fiber diets:

1. Arthritis
2. Cancer
3. Cholesterol elevations
4. Diabetes
5. Diverticulitis
6. Duodenal ulcer
7. Gallbladder disease
8. Gastric ulcer
9. Gout
10. Heart disease
11. Hemorrhoids
12. High blood pressure
13. Hypoglycemia
14. Inflammatory bowel
15. Obesity
16. Triglyceride elevation
17. Venous disease (varicose veins and blood clots)

Constipation, though not a disease in itself, is due primarily to a lack of fiber in the diet. It is one of the most common health maladies in America today. Most cases of constipation are cured simply by adding additional fiber to the diet. Be sure to increase water intake at the same time. For those stubborn cases where fiber alone doesn't do the job, a variety of remedies are listed on page 223.

SPECIAL FOODS FOR HEALTHY INTESTINES

Certain foods greatly activate the intestines, improving digestion and promoting elimination. A partial list includes:

- figs
- dates (fresh)
- peppers
- cabbage (raw)
- sauerkraut
- watermelon
- grapes (fresh)
- cucumbers (fresh)
- parsley (raw)
- beets with tops (fresh)
- ground flax seed
- turnips with tops (fresh)
- horseradish
- onions (raw)
- garlic
- radishes
- Jerusalem artichokes
- pears (fresh)

CANCER BEGINS IN THE MOUTH

Oral hygiene should be considered important by the dentist and physician alike. Unfortunately, many doctors fail to emphasize how critical proper dental hygiene really is.

The health of the oral cavity, the gums, and the teeth are related to the susceptibility to cancer. The healthier and stronger the gums and dentition are — the more free of disease they are — the less vulnerable an individual will be to cancer. You are probably wondering how this could be. There are several reasons why. As you may know, cancer is directly related to the health of the immune system. Infected teeth and gums stress immunity, and certain infections in the mouth can actually depress the immune system throughout the body. Second, chronic infections in the gums or roots of the teeth are directly related to the cause of certain cancers. In these instances, the chronic infections poison the immune system's central defenses. In essence, the immune system becomes paralyzed. Because of this, cancer can more easily gain a foothold. Third, the oral cavity, if healthy, prevents the spread of infection, acting as a guardian for the rest of the body. When its structural components such as the gums break down, whether due to nutritional deficiency, poor diet, excess sugar, or other stressors, existing infections within the mouth can spread to infect other tissues. If disease of the oral cavity exists, various microorganisms contracted through the environment can more easily gain a foothold. Remember, billions upon billions of microorganisms of all types live in the mouth — bacteria, fungi, yeasts, and viruses — many of which can cause disease. Even a slight imbalance within them can lead to ill-health.

Over 95% of Americans have gum disease, and most have had one or more cavities. Many factors play a role in creating this. Refined sugar, white flour, soft drinks, pastries and/or candy, if consumed regularly, are bound to cause gum disease. The consumption of excess quantities of soft drinks is associated with erosion of the enamel. This sets the stage for infections of the teeth themselves, known more commonly as cavities. Deficiencies of calcium, vitamin D, vitamin C, bioflavonoids, zinc, coenzyme Q-10 and folic acid are associated with gum disease.

Of major importance are the nutrients folic acid and coenzyme Q-10. It has been found that diseased gums contain much less of these two nutrients than healthy ones. Supplementation with coenzyme Q-10 and folic acid has proven to prevent gum disease and in some cases, even reverse the damage.

A new method for improving dental hygiene is available. It is called the Rota-dent, a device very similar to the rotating brush used by dentists to clean teeth professionally. Since keeping the teeth and gums clean is valuable to overall health, I usually recommend that patients with all varieties of diseases utilize some form of home dental hygiene. However, studies have shown that the Rota-dent is more effective than regular toothbrushing. In addition, it is at least as effective, if not more so, than a combination of brushing and flossing. In some instances, it may even eliminate the need for flossing. Research has shown that this unique device removes plaque and decreases the count of plaque-causing bacteria.

The Rota-dent is the perfect hygiene device for those interested in preventive dentistry. Regular use is likely to prevent the occurrence of chronic gum and root infections. Thus, there is the esthetic aspect of its use — healthier gums, whiter teeth and fresher breath. For more information contact:

ROTA-DENT
P.O. Box 12091
Des Moines, Iowa 50312

If you are ill, whether it be a result of arthritis, diabetes, peptic ulcer, colitis, chronic infection, or heart disease, your ailment may have much of its origin in the mouth. Cleaning up the health of your teeth and gums is likely to result in a noticeable improvement in how you feel. Improved oral hygiene is a critical component of cancer prevention.

YOUR WATER MAY BE CONSTIPATING YOU

Constipation is truly the plague of modern civilization. One-third or more of Americans have it. There is plenty of proof that those who are chronically constipated are more susceptible to cancer. Did you know that some types of water cause constipation? Namely, our chlorinated drinking water. Chlorine compounds in tap water kill the helpful intestinal bacteria, leading to an overgrowth of harmful bacteria, yeasts, or even parasites. In addition, tap water may itself contain parasites or their cysts. If you are easily constipated, you might be reacting to the water you drink.

What are the alternatives? The possibilities are many. It would be foolish to stop drinking water altogether. The simplest solution is to purify the water at its source. This subject is discussed at length later in this chapter. I do not recommend drinking distilled water, as it increases the excretion of valuable minerals. This includes cancer-protective minerals such as calcium, silicon, zinc and selenium.

TOXIC CHEMICALS AND CANCER

Toxic chemicals play a major role in the genesis of cancer. These chemicals are found within the food, water, air and soil. Some are added directly to food when it is processed. For example, the preservative BHT is added to corn oil. Another example is food dyes which are added to everything from Kool-Aid to pickles. Others are absorbed directly from the soil into the food or are found as residues on the food when crops are sprayed. Still other chemicals are ingested through drinking water. Our fresh water supplies are quickly becoming a toxic nightmare. They are laced with poisons and carcinogens, the result of industrial wastes, agricultural run-off, pesticides, herbicides, and radioactive chemicals which seep into ground water stores. Unfortunately, these wastes are accumulating faster than they can ever be removed.

OUR GRAIN IS CONTAMINATED - THE AFLATOXIN STORY

Natural chemicals can also contaminate the environment. Molds which grow on stored grain release several potent chemicals. Aflatoxin is one example. This poison is 100 times more potent in causing cancer than PCBs. PCBs are highly toxic synthetic chemicals made from the residues of coal and oil production.

Aflatoxin is the most powerful carcinogen known. The grain crop of 1988, especially the corn, was heavily contaminated with aflatoxin. Stored corn, already weakened by the drought, became infested with a fungus which releases aflatoxin in minute quantities. However, enough of the chemical got into the food chain through corn and cattle products to increase all of our cancer risks. For example, in Texas, millions of pounds of milk were dumped due to aflatoxin contamination, and it doesn't take much. Millionths of a gram can initiate precancerous or cancerous changes. This serious health threat was thoroughly exposed in the *Wall Street Journal* (February 23, 1989).

Unfortunately, government surveillance of aflatoxin contamination of grain, milk, or meat is inadequate despite laws in existence to protect the public from it. Dr. David Wilson of the University of Georgia was quoted by the Journal as stating that neither government nor industry were capable of dealing with the problem. Mr. R. Leonard of the Community Nutrition Institute in Washington D.C. says there will be more cancers over the next 10 to 20 years due to aflatoxin. The readers of this book can by-pass this dilemma by following the grain-free dietary guidelines, and by taking antioxidants as outlined in Chapter 6. People whose diet consists mostly of grains, such as wheat, corn, or rye probably have increased amounts of aflatoxin in their livers as well as in other tissues. For those who are concerned that they were or are being exposed, take high doses of vitamin E (1200 I.U.), beta carotene (75,000 I.U.), and selenium (400 to 600 mcg.) over the next year and all should be well. In addition, a recent scientific study published in 1988 has shown that certain minerals, most notably manganese, copper, and zinc as well as selenium, blocks the ability of aflatoxin to induce cancer. But most important, stay away from grains, especially corn and limit the consumption of milk.

Unfortunately, for many people there is no way to escape having some intake of aflatoxin. The food sources are many, and it is difficult, if not impossible, to avoid them all. In these cases, reliance must be placed on helping the body detoxify it through the antioxidant program outlined previously, and by taking substances known as *liver protectors*.

LIVER PROTECTORS — THE ANSWER TO TOXIC SCARES

The aflatoxin problem is not the first toxic scare to surface in the last 20 years. Chernobyl, Bhopal, Three Mile Island, and the U.S.A. dioxin contamination are some examples, just to name a few. Each time we are told of the potential or actual damage to human health these disasters cause. But do you ever remember being told that you can do something about it — that if these toxins reach you through food, air or water that you can protect yourself? Well, to a large degree you can — through liver protectors. In the case of aflatoxin poisoning, protection and treatment of the liver is of utmost importance since aflatoxin exerts its primary toxicity on liver cells and, thus, greatly increases the risks for liver cancer.

WHY PROTECT THE LIVER

It is of critical importance to protect the liver because it is the primary organ responsible for processing and removing toxic compounds. Well over 90% of the detoxification process for substances such as aflatoxin, dioxin, pesticides, and hydrocarbons occurs in the liver. These chemicals damage the liver and/or cause liver cancer, which is becoming more common in the U.S.A. every year. So it is important to give the liver cells double if not triple protection. The liver contains billions of cells, and in most of us, they are crying for more protection. The following are the liver protectors which can be used to beef-up your defenses.

Protector:
BEET JUICE WITH TOPS (fresh squeezed)

Comment:

Beets and beet tops contain special substances, some of which are yet to be identified which protect liver cells from damage. They also help heal liver cells once they are injured. Beets also contain a substance which stimulates the flow of bile, thus reducing liver congestion. Hepatitis, whether caused by viruses or chemicals often responds to beet juice. However, you have to drink at least a quart or more per day.

Protector:
CHLORELLA

Comment

This is an excellent protector, since it actually helps pull poisons out of the liver. This may be due in part to its high chlorophyll content. Chlorella also minimizes the toxin load on the liver by aggressively binding to a variety of harmful substances including cadmium, lead, mercury, pesticides, herbicides, and chlorinated hydrocarbons (PCBs, THMs, TCEs, etc.). It is likely that chlorella will remove aflatoxin as well.

Protector:
LIPOIC ACID

Comment

Lipoic acid actually seals off and stops damage to liver cells which have been exposed to toxic substances. It is the treatment of choice for certain types of mushroom poisoning — conditions which would otherwise be fatal.

It is useful in the treatment of most types of chemical hepatitis. Lipoic acid is available as *Thioctic*, made by Cardiovascular Research (see appendix B).

Protector:
BIOTIN

Comment

Whenever liver damage occurs, the liver cells swell and become infiltrated with fat. In order for these cells to recover quickly from any toxic insult, it is necessary to *get the fat out*. Biotin does this well. Its primary role as a B-vitamin is to modulate fat metabolism. At least 5 to 10 milligrams per day of biotin are needed to accomplish this. An excellent biotin (10 mg.) is made by GY&N Products (see appendix B).

Protector:
LIQUID GARLIC EXTRACT
(raw or cooked garlic also works, but to a lesser degree).

Comment

Garlic extracts formulated for medical use have been proven in many research studies to have a dramatic, protective effect on the liver. Improvement of the liver's ability to remove poisons, kill bacteria, parasites, or viruses, and to heal itself after chemical exposure has been documented. One study showed that a significant rise in liver content of glutathione peroxidase occurred following therapy with garlic extract. Glutathione peroxidase (GP), as described in Chapter 6, is the cells' front line of defense and the liver cells are no exception. In fact, the liver contains more GP that any other organ in the body. It is a good rule of thumb that, whenever the liver is stressed, its GP levels drop. The most valuable things I know of which raise GP levels are the antioxidants selenium and vitamin E, and garlic extract.

An excellent, clinically tested liquid garlic extract is made by the Wakunaga Corporation, under the brand name *SGP Garlic* (see appendix B). A good daily maintenance dose is 4 gelatin capsules daily, two in the morning and two at night. If you sustain a significant toxic exposure, double or even triple this dose.

Protector:
BIFIDOBACTERIA

Comment

The existence of harmful bacteria within the intestines is bad news for the liver. This is because the liver receives 80% of all blood flow from the intestines. No doubt, this blood carries vitamins, minerals, sugars, amino acids, and other nutrients to the liver where some of these substances are utilized. Yet, this blood also delivers all sorts of by-products resulting from bacterial fermentation within the intestines. The wrong kind of bacteria, if allowed to multiply in excess, will release substances which compromise the liver's ability to function. These bacteria can get into the blood stream and flow into the liver. The liver is set up to kill bacteria, since 30% of its weight is made up of cells somewhat similar to white blood cells (*Kuppfer cells*), which function to filter out foreign invaders. Even so, the added burden of these bacteria and the toxins they produce places tremendous stress upon the liver. This may be why people who regularly eat fermented milk products live such a long and healthy life, since these food products contain prodigious quantities of friendly bacteria (lactobacillus bifidus and acidophilus). These friendly bacteria act to "crowd out" the harmful ones, reducing their overall number and, thus, diminishing the toxic load on the liver. Bifidobacteria are also useful for inactivating cancer-causing chemicals found within the bowel before they travel to the liver. Believe me, a healthy liver means a long and healthy life.

In addition to consuming fermented milk products, friendly bacteria may be taken in supplemental form. Best results are achieved if both lactobacillus bifidus and acidophilus are taken, although I believe bifidobacteria to be the most important of the two. Several companies have made available high-quality bifidobacteria supplements, and the names include Klaire Labs (Vital-Plex), Metagenics (Ultrabifidus), and Wakunaga Corporation (Kyodophilus).

Protector:
CHOLINE (Lecithin)

Comment

For years it has been known that choline and other components of lecithin improve liver function. Lecithin is used by the liver to make bile and other fatty substances such as triglycerides. But more important, lecithin contains choline, which has been shown to protect liver cells from chemically-induced damage. In animals given cancer-causing chemicals, a deficiency of choline leads to pre-cancerous changes in their livers. When choline is added to the diet, these changes do not occur. Choline works best with a diet rich in high quality proteins such as eggs, fish, and meats. My favorite choline/lecithin supplement is *Supercholine*, made by Cardiovascular Research. It has higher amounts of choline per capsule than most lecithin supplements. To order:

Cardiovascular Research
1061-B Shary Circle
Concord, CA 94518
1-415-827-2636

With this product, a good maintenance dose is 2 capsules morning and night. For treating liver disease or toxicity, take a minimum of 3 to 4 capsules three times daily until symptoms dissipate, then return to the maintenance dosage.

Protector:
SILYMARIN

Comment

Silymarin is an herb from the milkweed family. Recently, much scientific research has shown that it protects the liver in particular from chemically-induced damage. Everyone living in the U.S.A. is receiving a daily dose of toxic chemicals. Less than 200 years ago, there was no such thing as a synthetic chemical. Now we are being exposed to thousands of them. The production of pesticides alone exceeds 1.4 billion pounds per year. Even a trace of pesticides is toxic to our bodies, and most of us are consuming much more than a trace. Today, Americans are experiencing some form of liver toxicity or damage as a result of these ubiquitous chemicals. A name can be coined for this condition — the Toxic American Liver Syndrome. Each day the liver must attempt to rid the body of a host of chemical poisons absorbed from the water, air, or food. For example, every minute it must deal with pesticides and herbicides from the food, chlorinated compounds and heavy metals from the water, and ozone and chloroform as well as other noxious gases from the air. This is why silymarin is so valuable. It protects liver cells from free radical damage, acting as an antioxidant. In fact its antioxidant activity, in terms of protecting the liver, greatly exceeds that offered by vitamin antioxidants such as beta carotene, vitamin C, and E.

The liver-healing effects of silymarin can be quite dramatic. Silymarin should be in your protector pharmacy *just in case*.

HYDROGENATED FATS AND POLYUNSATURATED OILS

The role refined fats play in cancer causation is becoming more understood with time. A definite increase in cancer risk is seen with the consumption of fats and oils, particularly all types of refined vegetable oils. Deep frying oils, most of which are hydrogenated, also contribute to this risk. In fact, it can be safely stated that the current American dietary practice of consuming refined fats and oils plays a greater role in causing cancer than any other single dietary factor. High quality cold-pressed oils and extra-virgin olive oil have not been correlated with increased risk. In fact, they may decrease the risks.

TOO MUCH IRON — A CANCER PROMOTER?

Now it is proven. There is such a thing as too much iron. It has been discovered that too much iron in the body increases the long-term risk for all types of cancer. Some of the best research on this subject is being done by Richard G. Stevens, PhD. He found that as little as a 3% rise in blood iron levels above the norm increased cancer risks in men by as much as 40%! This is an astonishing finding. Higher levels of iron further exaggerate the risks. Women did not show such a pattern. This is because their blood iron levels are consistently lower due to menstruation. However, the few women who did have excess levels of iron also had a higher rate of cancer.

Women who have no periods or who take the pill can also have excess iron. Women who have very light periods are also losing a smaller amount of iron.

I have consistently seen that cancer victims have a lot of iron in their blood. This finding has been confirmed by many cancer researchers. Yet, until recently, no one has discussed why excess iron predisposes to cancer.

EXCESS IRON DEPRESSES THE IMMUNE SYSTEM

Iron in excess is bad for health because it helps initiate a breakdown of the immune system. The presence of iron greatly enhances the rate at which damage can occur to the cells' most critical components — the genetic material. Iron somehow interacts with certain toxic molecules (remember the free radicals) to generate destructive chemical reactions. These reactions damage both the cell and its nucleus. Once the genes are repeatedly damaged, the cells can become cancerous. This is the same kind of thing which happens when a nuclear bomb drops or if there is a meltdown (as at Chernobyl).

When these reactions occur, they can penetrate all organs and cells in the body, although the cells of the immune system are particularly vulnerable. White blood cells are rapidly dividing cells; millions of them are made every hour. When they attack a microbe or detoxify a poison, hundreds of chemical reactions occur. In essence, they give off their own form of radiation. In the presence of iron, these reactions can backfire and actually kill the white cell. Having too much iron around inside our bodies is bad. It makes what are normal physiologic processes go haywire. Literally, these reactions go out of control. All sorts of cellular damage results. You can imagine the problems that will occur if immune cells are destroyed at a rate faster than they are made. Most certainly you will be left wide-open for all sorts of infections or even cancer.

CONTAMINATED WATER:
A MAJOR FACTOR IN CANCER CAUSATION

Unfortunately, our most valuable resource is being destroyed — our fresh water supply. Every well, river, or lake in the United States is polluted. In fact, the fresh water supplies throughout the world are now tainted with toxic chemicals, heavy metals, and other contaminants. Even the ice caps and icebergs contain measurable levels of these poisons. Are you concerned? You should be. Your cancer risks are greatly related to the degree to which your drinking water is polluted. In some regions the water is so toxic that one would be better off not to drink any water at all! Of course, each of us needs a certain amount of fluids. Water is essential to life. I am not suggesting that you totally curtail your fluid intake. What I am suggesting is that you do something to upgrade the water you drink.

WHAT YOU BATHE IN MAY BE HARMFUL TO YOUR HEALTH

You get more pollutants in your system through the water you drink than by direct contact, right? WRONG! Most people today are skimping on drinking tap water. Do you know anyone that has cut down on the number of baths or showers they are taking? You absorb more water through a bath or a 15 minute shower than it is likely you would drink in one day. Most people do not drink more than a quart of water per day. Immediately after taking a shower or bath, an individual can gain as much as three pounds. However, it is unlikely that there is any noticeable weight gain because the water evaporates very rapidly. But the toxic chemicals remain.

Let's look at this another way. For every 50 lbs. of body weight, up to one pound of water and impurities are absorbed. Thus, a person weighing 140 pounds would absorb over a quart of bath or shower water! The more you weigh, the more you will absorb. How is all of this water absorbed? Through the skin. The skin is like a sponge. It is the largest organ of the body and has an unbelievably large surface area. This is due to the innumerable tiny crevices and folds found on the skin. If spread out, it would cover an area the size of a tennis court or greater. Toxins from the water or environment can easily penetrate it. This poses a problem. When toxins enter our bodies through the digestive tract, they are confronted by cells of the immune system, which decompose and detoxify them. If toxins get past the immune cells, the liver siphons them out of the blood and attempts to rid us of them. However, direct absorption through the skin of harmful substances such as pesticides, herbicides, hydrocarbons, and heavy metals is often more damaging to our delicate immune systems than other means of exposure. A number of research studies have proven that the absorption of toxic chemicals through the skin is far more dangerous than a similar exposure through drinking water. Direct absorption through the skin of toxic substances can and has caused ill-health and even death.

PURIFYING YOUR WATER: WHAT ARE THE OPTIONS?

Most of you are now so concerned that you may stop drinking tap water entirely. I do not advise this. You need fluids daily to keep from dehydrating and to maintain proper kidney function. A better alternative is to drink tap water after removing any impurities. Water purification is a huge, multi-million dollar industry. Everyone from Sears to Culligan has jumped on the bandwagon. These next few pages will help you sort out fact from fiction so you can make the best choice possible in your attempt to improve the quality of the water you drink, shower, wash and/or bathe in.

DISTILLATION

In this process, water is heated to the point where it becomes steam. The steam, along with other vapors, including potentially toxic ones, go through some tubes where it condenses back to water. For example, chlorine in the water readily vaporizes into highly toxic chlorine gas when water is heated. Some toxic vapors remain in the water even after it is distilled. What is left behind is particulate matter, including impurities and all the minerals naturally contained in water.

Distillation is expensive and wasteful. A great deal of energy is used up in the process. But that is the least of the waste. Look at what is left behind. Yes, many impurities are removed, but so are the life-giving minerals such as calcium, magnesium, zinc, and selenium. It is bad enough that the food is depleted of these minerals. If you deplete the water too, you can really get into trouble. It is a fact that hard water rich in these and other minerals has an anti-cancer effect. We need all the cancer protection we can get. For this reason, I highly recommend *against* drinking distilled water.

REVERSE OSMOSIS

Reverse osmosis water purifiers are wasteful in a different way. It takes eight gallons of water to make *one* gallon of purified water. That's right! Eight gallons go down the drain. I do not believe our limited resources of fresh water can withstand such waste. Fresh water makes up only 3% of the total water on the earth. Fully 2% of this is locked up in glacial ice, the north and south poles, and icebergs. In fact, less than 1/4 of 1% of all the water in the world is available for human use. Can you imagine the problems that could result if everyone used such a wasteful method?

In addition, some reverse osmosis purifiers utilize sodium and, in many instances, a residue of sodium is left in the water. All types of reverse osmosis units remove the more valuable minerals such as calcium, potassium, and magnesium. The following is an example of the ill-effects which occur from drinking water treated with reverse osmosis.

CASE HISTORY:
Magnesium deficiency likely due to drinking reverse osmosis water.

Mrs. J. was plagued with a history of repeatedly injuring her muscles and ligaments. At the slightest strain, such as picking up a bag of groceries or opening a jar lid, she would injure herself.

I suspected magnesium deficiency, since its lack leads to the muscles being easily injured and torn. Mrs. J. had one of the lowest blood magnesium levels I had ever seen. Not to my surprise, she had been religiously drinking only reverse osmosis water for over four years. This habit was the likely cause of her systemic magnesium deficiency.

WATER SOFTENERS

Water softeners are a form of reverse osmosis. They function by activating sodium molecules, turning them into *ions*. These ions go about "eating up" or destroying the other minerals in water which are responsible for its taste and hardness. The sodium ions destroy naturally occurring minerals in the water — just think of what they will do to the minerals in your body!

The use of softened water is highly correlated with an increased incidence of cancer, heart attacks, and strokes. Don't waste your water or health by drinking softened water.

BOTTLED WATER

Now you probably suspect what I am leading up to. Bottled water from the French Alps, right? Wrong! I believe that the only truly natural way to drink water is to drink *running water*. Stagnant water of any type, whether it is bottled under the most sterile conditions or it is in a fetid pond, is not water as nature intended it. Running water which undergoes all the natural processes is the best way to go. Water that originates as rain or snow, percolating from the ground — filtering through the many layers of rock and soil from which it absorbs and carries minerals — this is ideal. I realize that the ideal is not always possible, and in this respect, some of the higher quality bottled waters might be acceptable. But how do you know which ones are truly high-grade?

"BOTTLE WATER FIZZLES OUT"
SO SAYS THE WATER QUALITY ASSOCIATION

In 1987, this respected organization tested bottled water found on the shelves of New York City's supermarkets. Increasingly, they found that 96% of the bottled water tested *worse* for chemicals and bacteria than did water from the tap! This proves my point. Bottled water is becoming a huge and highly competitive industry. Not everyone is as careful as you might think, and though that sealed bottle of water might *look* pure, it is likely laced with all kinds of contaminants, and possibly even bacteria and parasites.

TAP WATER PURIFIERS: THE LOGICAL SOLUTION

I would not take you through this journey without providing you with some answers. Tap water is far from perfect. It contains both good and bad elements. The bad elements, however, can be addressed effectively through in-house water filtration and purification units. This is especially important for those who bathe or shower frequently. The finest purifiers are those which remove toxic substances *including* the *chlorine* while allowing the health-giving minerals to pass through. It is important to retain as much calcium, magnesium, silicon, and selenium in the water as is possible. These minerals exert powerful protection against heart disease, arthritis, cancer, as well as other illnesses. In addition, these minerals, once dissolved in water, are readily absorbed by the body. This is because water acts as a solvent, causing the minerals to be ionized. Once in this state, the minerals are readily absorbed by the body.

A water treatment unit called the *Waterfier* has recently become available. This unit effectively removes toxic and potentially cancer-causing chemicals from the water. According to tests performed at the University of North Carolina, it also removes over 90% of the heavy metals, such as lead and cadmium, while allowing the critical trace elements to pass through. This is due in part to the fact that the Waterfier contains a unique form of carbon known as Bone-Char, which is extremely effective at binding lead, cadmium, mercury, aluminum, and other heavy metals.

This unit uses three systems of purification. They are fine filtration, activated carbon, and magnetization, all of which assist in the removal of impurities. No harmful chemicals or residues are added to the water in the process. An additional benefit is that, after treatment with the Water-fier, the water noticeably improves in taste and odor. Those owning their own home would be well advised to contact the purveyors of the Waterfier in respect to their whole-house water treatment units. It would be difficult to compare the value of such a unit for your home versus, for example, a new set of kitchen cabinets or some new furniture. To me, there is no com-parison between these. Health is not an exchangeable commodity. There is no way to put a dollar figure on health. More information about the Waterfier is available by contacting:

O'MARA PRECISION BUILDERS
3130 Eugene Street
Burton, Michigan 48519
1-313-743-8050

Unfortunately apartment dwellers and renters are not usually able to install household purifiers. However, they can still adequately clean up their water. Many countertop models are available on the market. It is easy to get confused in this area due to the wide selection available and the variations in price. The Waterfier countertop and under-the-sink models may be your best choice overall. Here are the reasons why:

1. To be safe and effective, countertop units must contain a mechanism for back-flushing. This is to prevent the build-up and growth of microorganisms within the carbon. Carbon, being organic, can be a medium for microbial growth and this does occur occasionally. This can be a hidden danger and most countertop units cannot be back-flushed. The Waterfier water treatment units, whether household, countertop, under-the-sink, or industrial, all contain back-flushing mechanisms.

2. The carbon in your water unit should be loose, not pressed. Most water treatment units contain either carbon blocks or loose carbon which is tightly packed. This leads to a phenomenon known as channeling. This means that channels actually form within the carbon matrix. When water passes through these channels, effective filtration is reduced significantly.

3. Activated carbon purifies water much like nature does through top soil or sand. Water within deep wells or aquafers gets purified by percolating through thousands of acres of top soil, silt, rock, and sand. This phenomenon is known as surface area contact. Activated carbon has a tremendous surface area for contacting and holding on to pollutants such as chlorinated hydrocarbons, pesticides, herbicides,

PCBs, THMs, TCE, benzene, gasoline and many similar compounds. One pound of carbon has the same water filtration capacity in terms of surface area as 112 acres of topsoil!

The key to taking advantage of this tremendous filtration capacity is that the water must have ample contact time with the carbon. Thus, if the water runs through the carbon too fast as is the case with most water treatment units, less poisons will be removed. The Waterfier allows for ample contact time to capitalize on the removal of the pollutants.

Pure water means better health. Every river, lake, stream, and well in this country is contaminated. With one out of three Americans developing cancer at some point in life, it is *life-threatening* not to purify your water. It makes little sense to "go all out" and eat pure, wholesome foods while drinking water which is full of toxic substances. Our water is contaminated with everything from parasites and pesticides to gasoline. Don't be fooled. The water in this country is getting worse by the day. Soon, water will be the most precious commodity on this earth. What you drink is every bit as important as what you eat. When seeking preventive health care, try to cover as many basis as possible. Proper dental hygiene, pure water, clean air, and nutritious foods are all important. Reducing or eliminating any contact with water-borne toxic chemicals is a big step in the right direction.

THE ROLE OF STRESS

Do you know of anyone whose cancer came on after a period of severe mental stress? Actually, this is most commonly what happens. In these cases, the genetic tendency for cancer often already exists.Yet, it is more often than not that severe emotional or psychological stress stimulates the growth of the cancer.

Stress has a negative effect upon the nervous system. The nervous system controls the function of the immune system. Stress or negative emotions such as anger, guilt or depression, can be transmitted along the nerve pathways ultimately leading to immune depression. An immunity already compromised by toxic chemicals, heavy metals, poor diet, and nutritional deficiency may be pushed over the limit by a prolonged period of stress. Even a relatively brief episode of stress, if severe enough, can precipitate the onset of cancer.

It may be argued that there already was an underlying cancerous tumor and the stress just served to hasten it to the surface. This may indeed be true. Yet, many of these individuals have been sensitive to the ill-effects of stress possibly for a lifetime. The role played by stress in the causation of cancer is so great that it would not be an exaggeration to say that 80% or more cancer cases have their immediate origin in some form of mental pressure or strain. Grief, distress, fear, worry and anger are emotions which have horrible effects on the body's functions. Researchers have discovered that these emotions cause the release of chemicals from the brain called neuropeptides. These potent compounds have a profound immune-suppressive action. Scientists have traced a pathway from the brain to the immune cells proving that negative emotions can stop the immune cells dead in their tracks. This results in part from the release of chemicals from nerve endings. Once this happens, harmful microbes or cancer cells can invade any tissue in the body.

The moral of this story is to be careful of what thoughts you allow yourself to entertain. If you suspect that negative thought patterns are circulating in your mind, patterns which are having a detrimental effect upon your health, it is possible to change them. By changing your thoughts from negative (minus) to positive (plus), your health will change for the better. Disease indicates the need for change. No one can change the situation better than you. For some, this may be the best cancer prevention of all.

NUTRITIONAL DEFICIENCIES AND CANCER
SELENIUM DEFICIENCY

This mineral is a key factor in cancer prevention. Regions with the highest soil and water concentrations of selenium have the lowest cancer incidence. The Great Lakes region (Wisconsin, Illinois, Indiana, Michigan, and Ohio) has one of the highest cancer rates in the world. As you may have guessed, this region has virtually no selenium in its soil. Many coastal states also have selenium-deficient soil, particularly those in the Northeastern and Northwestern regions.

Selenium activates an enzyme in the body known as glutathione peroxidase. Its function is to protect cell membranes, genetic material, and the immune system from damage due to toxic chemicals, heavy metals, radiation, and stress. Without selenium, this enzyme becomes powerless to protect you.

When selenium or glutathione deficient cells are bombarded with cancer-causing substances, their genetic material goes haywire and this is the beginning of cancer. This is because the genes control the rate at which cells reproduce. A tumor is essentially cellular reproduction gone out of control. Selenium may well be the most important cancer-protective nutrient known.

BETA CAROTENE

This nutrient has been proven to be instrumental in preventing cancer. Research is now showing that beta carotene actually helps the body destroy tumor cells. The activity of special anti-tumor cells known as macrophages is greatly increased by supplemental and/or dietary beta carotene. In addition, beta carotene itself is directly toxic to certain tumors. Beta carotene is found primarily in vegetables, tubers (root plants), and fruits. Rich food sources include:

alfalfa leaves
apricots
asparagus
avocados
beet tops
broccoli
butter
cantaloupe
carrots
chard, Swiss
chili peppers
chlorella
collards
dandelion greens
endive
escarole

green onions
kale
mustard greens
parsley
persimmons
pimentos
pumpkin
red peppers
romaine lettuce
spinach
sweet potatoes
tomatoes
turnip greens
turnips
watercress
winter squash
yellow squash

NATIONAL CANCER INSTITUTE AND BETA CAROTENE

For several years now, the NCI as well as the American Cancer Society have recommended that diets include foods rich in beta carotene. They know that the evidence is clear: diets enriched with foods such as those mentioned above prevent cancer. Take heed of this and include prodigious quantities of these foods in your diet. A good rule of thumb is to snack on beta carotene-rich vegetables every day in addition to including them with your meals.

HOW BETA CAROTENE WORKS

Beta carotene exerts its protective effect in a number of ways. It directly protects cells from the damaging ions generated in the body due to radiation. People receiving x-rays should greatly increase their beta carotene consumption. Beta carotene also enhances the body's ability to utilize oxygen at the cellular level. If the oxygen concentration within the cells is high enough, cancer cannot develop.

The loss of the earth's ozone layer is allowing more radioactive particles to penetrate the atmosphere. These extra ions are also penetrating our bodies. Once these ions enter the body, they cause damaging reactions which can destroy the nuclear material (genes and chromosomes) within the cells. Beta carotene blocks these reactions. By increasing the consumption of beta carotene-rich foods, it is possible to decrease the degree of damage to the body caused by the sun's radioactive waves. For an added protective effect, I recommend supplementing your diet with a potent, natural source of beta carotene such as carrot juice, chlorella, or beta carotene extract. I do not recommend synthetic beta carotene.

BETA BOOSTER

A quick and simple way to get your beta carotene is to use the "Beta Booster." Simply mix one packet of chlorella granules with 8 oz. of fresh or canned carrot juice. This will satisfy your beta carotene needs for about 2 days. If you are getting a lot of radiation or toxic chemical exposure, you can use the Beta Booster daily. To improve the absorption of beta carotene, you may add 2 to 4 ounces of aloe vera juice. I recommend the MPS-fortified (i.e. MucoPolySaccharide) variety only (see appendix B).

VITAMIN E

Cancer patients are often deficient in vitamin E. Does this mean cancer is caused by vitamin E deficiency, or that it can be cured by it? Not really. All it means is that vitamin E helps protect the body against cancerous degeneration. Vitamin E in doses up to 1200 I.U. has a stimulating action on immune function. White blood cells which contain adequate quantities of vitamin E are able to survive longer and are more effective in killing foreign invaders, including cancer cells. It also helps by conserving other antioxidants such as glutathione, selenium, and coenzyme Q-10.

VITAMIN C

This vitamin offers its most potent anti-cancer actions when it is consumed in fresh fruits and vegetables. Much ado has been generated in regard to the beneficial effects of vitamin C supplements upon cancer. No doubt, vitamin C is a critical nutrient for assisting immune function. Even so, there is no solid evidence that supplements of synthetic vitamin C, whether powder or pills has any curative or anti-tumor action in respect to existing tumors. On the other hand, studies have shown that regular consumption of vitamin C-rich foods, such as fresh citrus fruits, greatly diminishes the incidence of cancer. This protective effect may not be from the vitamin C per se, but from a combined action of vitamin C, bioflavonoids, pigments, citrus oils, and other naturally occurring components in the whole fruit (including the fiber).*

*Vitamin C as a nutritional supplement is useful in a variety of other conditions, and it does help enhance immune function in the case of colds, flu, and other infections.

FISH OILS

Fish may well be brain food. Did you know it is also immune food? Fish oils have an anti-tumor action. They exert this effect primarily by preventing the spread of cancer into the tissues. Fish oils may also help block the formation of tumors.

The chemical name for fish oils is *eicosapentaenoic acid* (EPA) and *docosahexaenoic acid* (DHA). Their actions may be due in part to the dramatic improvement in circulation they cause. Fish oils decrease the sludging of blood, acting as a natural blood thinner. Cancer often spreads to other tissues through the blood. Cancer cells usually ride along on platelets, which carry them from their primary site to more distant sites throughout the body. Fish oils, by decreasing the stickiness of platelets, help stop this from happening. Another desirable effect is that they improve circulation. This leads to an increase in the oxygen content of the blood. Cancer cells grow best when the tissue oxygen concentration is low.

Also, it has been discovered that fish oils directly enhance the function of white blood cells, making them more effective in fighting infection and destroying malignant cells. A world of caution: only high quality fish oils exert this protective effect. The best source would be eating fish rich in EPA and DHA, although fish oil supplements are also helpful. EPA/DHA-rich fish include salmon, tuna, whitefish, sardines, trout, mackerel, and herring.

FOODS THAT IMPROVE THE ODDS

Diet has a lot to do with cancer risk. What you eat can either improve or worsen the odds. What you drink makes a difference too. The two categories of foods offering the highest degree of protection are fruits and vegetables. Cultures which have a high intake of fresh fruits and vegetables have a low cancer incidence. In some societies with extraordinary high intakes, cancer is literally non-existent. Let's examine some of the reasons why.

THE WONDER OF FRUITS

Fruits are good for you. There are a number of reasons why. First, they are highly digestible. The digestive organs put out far less energy to digest fresh fruits than to process, for instance, a piece of bread or a slice of roast beef. Fruits are loaded with anti-cancer substances. A word of caution: only fresh fruits provide these benefits. Fruits which are picked unripe, stored, fumigated, and waxed, or which are laden with pesticides or herbicides, are not likely to have cancer-protective benefits. Unfortunately, this is the case with most of our fresh fruit. Thus, the following information holds true only if fruits are fresh and free of contamination.

Protective Effects

There are many fruits which help protect us from getting cancer. For example, people living in citrus-growing regions such as Florida who eat large quantities of fresh citrus fruits have a lesser incidence of intestinal and stomach cancer. Citrus fruits are a rich source of two key nutrients: vitamin C and bioflavonoids. Both inactivate toxic or cancer-causing chemicals. They also protect our bodies from the harmful effects of these chemicals. Researchers have shown that a diet high in fresh citrus fruit leads to a reduction in the amount of cancer-causing chemicals, known as *mutagens,* in the feces.

In addition, bioflavonoids and vitamin C help keep the cellular cement in place. The cells in our body are bound to each other by connective tissue which is, in essence, microscopic ligaments. Vitamin C is required for the synthesis of these connective tissues, and bioflavonoids plug the gaps, acting as a sort of cellular glue. Vitamin C is needed on a continual basis to keep the bonds tight and prevent the glue from breaking down. In this way, vitamin C and bioflavonoids help prevent the invasion and spread of cancer. The tighter the "fit" of the cells, the more difficult it is for tumors to grow, invade, or metastisize.

An extreme example of breakdown in the cellular cement is scurvy. This vitamin C and bioflavonoid deficiency disease is becoming more common and not just in alcoholics or the elderly. In this condition, the gaps between cells and within cell membranes are so extensive that the body becomes invaded by all sorts of toxins, infections, and tumors. Cancer itself may be a form of a scurvy-like disease due to the degeneration of the connective tissues.

People who crave fruits are likely deficient in vitamin C. Those who crave the rinds of citrus fruits or who love to suck on lemons or limes usually have a deficiency of bioflavonoids. Rich food sources of each are listed below:

VITAMIN C

black currants
broccoli
Brussels sprouts
cantaloupe
cauliflower
citrus fruits (all types)
elderberries
green and red peppers (raw)
guava
hot peppers
juices - unsweetened citrus, papaya,
     strawberry, cranberry and tomato
kale
kiwi fruit
lamb's quarter
mustard greens
papaya
parsley (raw)
pimento
potatoes
red cabbage
spinach
strawberries
tomatoes (vine-ripened)
turnip greens
watercress
watermelon

BIOFLAVONOIDS

alfalfa
apricots
blackberries
black currants
broccoli
buckwheat
cantaloupe
cherries
citrus pulp
citrus rind
elderberries
grapes
green peppers
herbal teas (especially those
    containing rose hips)
plums
pure, raw vinegars
red onions
strawberries
tangerine juice

Here are three excellent, simple ways to get your daily dose of bioflavonoids:

1. Douse your salad with raw vinegar. Doctor Bronner's grape vinegar or Hain raw apple cider vinegar are excellent choices. Other good brands are found in specialty shops, health food stores, and some supermarkets.

2. Drink one or more cups daily of herbal tea containing rose hips or other flower buds.

3. Drink fresh-squeezed tangerine, grapefruit or orange juice every day. Tangerine is an exceptionally good source.

Bioflavonoids can help as a part of your cancer-protection armamentarium. They are also useful in treating and preventing the following conditions:

1. anemia (due to blood loss)
2. bleeding gums
3. bruising
4. diabetes
5. easy bruising
6. glaucoma (certain types)
7. heavy menstrual bleeding
8. hemorrhoids
9. miscarriage
10. phlebitis (blood clots)
11. stomach or intestinal ulcers
12. urinary bleeding
    (if not due to a tumor)
13. uterine fibroids
14. varicose veins

VITAMIN C IN FRUITS INACTIVATES CARCINOGENS

Foods rich in vitamin C preserve the health of the tissues. Just how vitamin C acts as a natural preservative is best illustrated by some common observations. Once a food is cut open, it rapidly loses its vitamin C content. As the vitamin C disappears, the food becomes susceptible to oxidation which is represented by loss of taste as well as color changes. A good example of this reaction is what happens to a banana or potato when they are peeled — they turn brown. This is the process of oxidation in action. It results from rapid loss of vitamin C into the air.

Toxins and carcinogens (cancer-causing chemicals) cause our tissues to oxidize, and vitamin C prevents this reaction from occurring. In addition, vitamin C can actually help the body destroy harmful chemicals. Meats preserved with nitrates are a good example. Nitrates, as described in Chapter 5, are chemicals used in the production of processed and cured meals. Examples of foods processed with nitrates include: hot dogs, bologna, bacon, sausage, ham, pastrami and corned beef. Nitrates are responsible for the bright reddish color of these meats. Thus, nitrates are used both for preservation and consumer appeal. However, the very thing manufacturers use to cure these meats acts as a powerful cancer-initiating substance once it is ingested. You can visualize the harmful effects of nitrates as actually "curing" your innards! Here is where vitamin C enters the picture. Substantial doses will block the toxicity of nitrates, and stop them from producing their most harmful effect — cancer. In fact, cured meats are associated with a significant increase in the incidence of cancer of the esophagus, intestines and stomach. Ironically, vitamin E, as a meat preservative, is just as effective as are nitrates but without the toxicity.

FRUITS IN THE GROCERY STORE
MAY NOT BE AS FRESH
AS THEY APPEAR

That's right, looks can be deceiving. Sometimes you can tell that the fruit is picked green; note the major difference in color, texture and shape of store-bought tomatoes versus the tomatoes grown in a garden. A similar, measurable difference occurs in the nutrient content as well. When a fruit is allowed to ripen naturally on a tree or vine, the nutrient content increases dramatically. This is due to the interaction between sunlight and the fruit. During the ripening process, sunlight is needed to cause chemical reactions within the fruit, resulting in an increased concentration of nutrients. This increased nutrient content is the major reason why fruits ripened on the tree or vine taste so much better. On the other hand, prolonged storage, gas-induced ripening, waxing, and fumigation all lead to the loss of delicate nutrients such as vitamin C, magnesium, potassium, chromium, manganese, vitamin E, and beta carotene.

ORANGES WITHOUT VITAMIN C, ANYONE?

In some instances, eating a "fresh" orange from the supermarket gives you no more vitamin C than eating a plastic one. At the Rockefeller Institute, Dr. Michael Colgan showed that some oranges found on the supermarket shelves actually scored zero in vitamin C content.

What can you do about it? Not much. Fruits in season are more reliable in their nutrient content. Certainly, if you have access to organically-grown fruits, this would be a good option. Do not be entirely discouraged. Many fruits retain their vitamin C content despite all the abuse they receive. A partial list of such fruits includes:

avocado   cranberries
kiwi fruit   strawberries
lemons   melons
limes   papaya

VEGETABLES

Vegetables may be the finest food category for the prevention of cancer. There are many reasons why. The fact that most vegetables are rich in three of the most effective anti-cancer nutrients known is of major importance. These are beta carotene, chlorophyll, and fiber.

Vegetables are a stress-free food. By this I mean they are easy to digest. Very little effort or energy is required by the digestive tract to process them. Proteins, on the other hand, require much more energy to be broken down into an absorbable form.

Vegetables are also non-putrifying. This means that few, if any, toxic by-products are produced in the intestines as a result of their digestion. Be sure to include a healthy portion of fresh vegetables in your diet on a daily basis. This is the best cancer prevention advice I can give.

RAW VERSUS COOKED VEGETABLES

Contrary to what some health advocates advise, not all vegetables need to be eaten raw. Sometimes steaming your vegetables, sauteing lightly in butter or olive oil, or even simmering them in a small amount of water, can be even better than eating them raw. If broccoli, cauliflower and Brussels sprouts are lightly cooked they provide far more nutrition than if they are eaten raw. You will get this message by seeing how much more vibrant and intense their colors appear once they are gently steamed or sauteed. Thus, for certain vegetables, cooking serves to activate the nutrients, making them easier to digest and assimilate.

Some vegetables appear to have a more potent cancer-preventive effect than others. A good case in point are those of the cabbage family —the *cruciferous* vegetables. This family includes cabbage, Brussels sprouts, cauliflower, broccoli, mustard greens, brown mustard, watercress and kohlrabi. Research has shown that these vegetables contain natural chemicals which block the formation of tumors in the stomach, colon, and rectum. A more recent study documented how cruciferous plants can even stop the spread of cancer once it is established!

Cabbage itself is known to exert a highly protective action against diseases of the stomach including stomach cancer. Along with the other vegetables in its family, cabbage also protects against the occurrence of breast cancer.

You may be curious why these vegetables are so powerful in preventing cancer. Nature was indeed generous in providing them for our use. We do not yet know all the reasons why they are so effective. Obviously, they contain their own unique group of chemicals which are highly specific in anti-cancer activity. In addition, cruciferous plants are rich in antioxidants such as vitamin C, selenium, and beta carotene. Regardless of the reason, the research is in. Add them to your diet freely and in large quantities — a piece of advice for peace of mind.

A LITTLE CHLOROPHYLL
WITH YOUR VEGETABLES, ANYONE?

Chlorophyll is found in all types of vegetation. It serves as the blood of the plant. Just as our blood is red (hemoglobin is our molecular equivalent to chlorophyll), the blood of plants is green. Chlorophyll exerts powerful anti-cancer protection. It helps prevent the build-up of potentially cancer-causing compounds by inactivating them and carrying them out of the system. In addition, it is a rich source of naturally occurring magnesium, needed by all cells in the body for their proper health.

Chlorophyll-rich vegetables include parsley, watercress, alfalfa, spinach, broccoli, and other dark greens. The richest known source of chlorophyll is chlorella. This single-celled, fresh water algae far exceeds other vegetation in chlorophyll content and, thus, can be used as a supplemental source.

STRIKE GOLD WITH YELLOW AND ORANGE VEGETABLES

Vegetables and tubers with a deep yellow or orange color are some of the richest sources of beta carotene in the world. These include pumpkin, squash, carrots, and sweet potato. Their bright yellow and orange colors are due to the heavy concentration of carotene pigments.

A nice addition to your diet would be pumpkin soup. You can make any of your favorite soups rich in beta carotene by adding diced pumpkin, squash or carrots. Sweet potatoes, if you can handle the starch and calories, would make an excellent snack or dinner addition.

SPECIAL VEGETABLES FOR SPECIAL PEOPLE

You are a very special person. Your body has a right to be cared for. Cancer is an invasion of your inner privacy. It can be an invasion of your rights. A good example of this is cancer in a teen-ager resulting from exposure to the estrogenic drug DES while in the womb. DES and many other cancer-causing chemicals have been used extensively in the food chain. There are thousands of other chemicals being used on our foods, even though they haven't been shown to be safe. On the contrary, many of them have been proven to be deleterious. Eating copious amounts of vegetables listed in the following special category can be instrumental in preventing this invasion:

broccoli	Brussels sprouts
cabbage	carrots
cauliflower	cucumber
garlic	kale
kohlrabi	mustard greens
onions	parsley
pumpkin	red peppers
squash	turnip greens
watercress	zucchini

GARLIC — NATURE'S #1 ANTI-CANCER SUBSTANCE

A perusal of cancer-preventive foods and herbs could not be complete without a discussion about garlic. Garlic has been used as a remedy for a wide range of ailments for centuries. Lately, there is much interest in the use of garlic therapeutically in relation to its positive effects upon the immune system. It seems that garlic contains a number of compounds which improve immune function. Here is a list of some of garlic's immune-enhancing properties as discovered by researchers in the last decade:

1. Inhibits the growth of tumor cells in test tubes.

2. Prevents chemically-induced stomach and colon cancer.

3. Prevents skin cancer induced by the chemical dimethyl benzanthracene.

4. Causes the destruction of bladder tumors in animals (by injecting garlic extract directly into the tumor)

5. Increases the activity of white blood cells, improving their ability to destroy tumor cells.

6. Helps increase the production of antibodies by B-lymphocytes.

7. Increases the activity of white blood cells in the human body known as *killer cells*, whose function is to destroy cancer cells.

8. Improves the function of the skin's immune system.

9. Increases body stores of the antioxidants glutathione and selenium.

10. Destroys harmful microorganisms which depress the immune system.

Why does garlic have all these positive effects? The answers are not all in. Garlic is one of the richest dietary sources of selenium, a mineral critical in maintaining immune defenses. It is also rich in glutathione and other sulfur-containing compounds. These compounds benefit the immune system in a variety of ways. In addition, garlic is directly toxic to cancerous tumors as well as to certain microbes, such as fungi, yeasts, and even certain viruses.

Garlic provides benefits whether it is raw, cooked, or taken in a supplemental form. It is not a good idea to eat excessive quantities of raw garlic. A clove a day or every other day would be more than sufficient. Larger doses can be taken if the garlic is cooked or in the form of an extract (see appendix B).

While I am not promoting garlic as a cure for cancer, I am insisting that it is the number one food for preventing it. When possible, get garlic which is fresh or organically grown. Commercial garlic is irradiated, a process which destroys some of its useful properties.

SUMMARY

Three out of every four households have been or will be hit by cancer. Those who have experienced the physical and mental trauma that it causes understand the following facts:

1. that cancer, once it develops, is difficult to treat and cure

2. that cancer often leads to a slow, painful death

3. that often, much mental and emotional trauma strikes both the cancer victim and his/her loved-ones

4. that, at this time, there are no known cures for cancer

With these facts, it is obvious that there is only one simple solution — preventing cancer from ever developing. This can be done. It is being done in many civilizations besides ours, where people eat wholesome foods rich in protective and immune-enhancing nutrients. Although we Americans have the added burden of a toxic, polluted environment, we also have the luxury of being able to double up on protective nutrients by taking nutritional supplements, and by having a wide variety of nutritious foods available.

CHAPTER 9
What About Food Allergies?

Wholesome foods are good for you, right? This is true as long as you are not allergic to them. In addition to the harmful foods, some of which have already been mentioned, even some naturally good foods could be bad for you. Throughout this book, you have been told that you couldn't go wrong with natural, unprocessed foods. However, this does not take into account the fact that you are probably allergic to several perfectly wholesome foods, which otherwise should be a part of your diet. But since I hate to see you get sick from eating things which seem good for you, I think we should delve into this a bit further. In fact, the right diet cannot be designed for you without knowing just what your food allergies are, since each person's set of allergies are unique.

YOUR UNIQUE SET OF FOOD ALLERGIES

No one knows exactly why each individual has his/her own distinct set of allergies. Sometimes the reasons can be determined. A common cause is food cravings which lead to the overeating of a certain food for a prolonged period of time. Eventually, an allergy to the food develops. Other allergies may develop early in life and can persist to a degree into adulthood. Some food allergies can even be inherited. However, no one knows for sure why one person is allergic, say to wheat, while another is allergic to oats or rye.

Regardless of the cause, many of the symptoms you may have are likely due to food allergies. Even if you do not have noticeable symptoms, it is likely that you are allergic to several foods. In addition, many diseases can be aggravated by continual exposure to allergic foods.

THE GREAT MIMICKER

Probably the most prevalent cause of symptoms which mimic other diseases is food allergies. A partial list of the symptoms they cause includes:

abdominal pain
anxiety
arrhythmia
back pain
bed wetting
bloating
burning eyes
burping
canker sores
chest pain (non-cardiac)
chills
chronic cough
colitis
confusion
cracked eyelids
cracked skin
crying spells
diarrhea
dizziness
earaches
ear discharge
eczema
eye discharge
fainting spells
fatigue
fever blisters
flatulence (gas)
flu-like symptoms
fluid retention
food cravings
gagging
headaches
hives

hoarseness
hunger pains
hyperactivity
indigestion
itchy ears
itchy mouth
itchy skin
irritability
joint aches
memory loss
mood swings
muscle aches
muscle twitching
neck pain
palpitations
ringing in ears
runny nose
salt cravings
shortness of breath
sleepiness
sneezing spells
sore throat
stomach pain
sweats
swollen ankles (or feet)
swollen eyelids
swollen fingers
urinary frequency
urinary urgency
violent behavior
weight gain
vaginal discharge

If you have 5 or more of these symptoms, it is possible that you have food allergies. If you have 10 or more, then food allergies are likely the cause of some of your symptoms. People who have 20 or more of these symptoms usually have multiple food allergies, and certain illnesses can result if these allergic foods are not eliminated.

ALLERGIES *CAN* PREDISPOSE TO DISEASE

Did you know that certain diseases can be caused or aggravated by the foods you eat? Intolerance to eggs, for example, could lead to a gallbladder attack. Sensitivity to pork or pork products can cause arthritis. Citrus fruits, especially oranges, may irritate the bladder and predispose to bladder infections. Wheat allergy predisposes certain people to colon or breast cancer. Allergy to aspirin compounds can cause or worsen asthma. Mold allergy often results in lung irritation which could lead to bronchitis or even pneumonia. Here is a partial list of diseases often having a food allergy component:

- Alzheimer's disease
- Arthritis
- Asthma
- Breast cancer
- Bronchitis
- Colon cancer
- Diabetes
- Diverticulitis
- Eczema
- Hardening of the arteries
- Heart disease
- High blood pressure
- Hypoglycemia
- Lupus
- Obesity
- Osteoarthritis
- Pancreatitis
- Parkinson's disease
- Peptic ulcer
- Psoriasis
- Psychosis
- Rectal cancer
- Rheumatoid arthritis
- Schizophrenia
- Stomach cancer
- Ulcerative colitis

A TIME WHEN BUTTER IS NOT BETTER

Here is an important concept: butter is better than margarine, right? Butter is natural, while margarine is synthetic. While this is true, there is a quirk. Butter is not better if you are allergic to it! If this be the case, I would recommend neither butter nor margarine. Olive or flax seed oil can replace butter for cooking purposes.

FOOD ALLERGY TESTING

One of the most accurate food allergy tests is the *Food Intolerance Test* performed through Nutritional Testing Laboratories. This test has an accuracy of 78%, far greater than scratch (30%) or Rast (5-10%) testing. It is easy to perform, requiring only a single tube of blood. Over 200 foods and food additives are tested. It is true that no allergy test is 100% accurate. Yet the value of this test is so great that I rarely begin dietary recommendations without it. You can imagine why. Think how awful a patient would feel and how embarrassed I would be if I recommended eating whole wheat bread in the event of a severe wheat allergy.

Once your food intolerances have been determined, I usually recommend the following course of action:

1. Stay off of all foods you are allergic to for at least 90 days

2. Stay off of all foods to which you are known to have had severe allergic reactions to during your childhood. These may not show up in the test, since it is likely that you have diligently avoided eating them.*

3. Re-introduce the allergic foods one at a time and keep track of the symptoms they produce. If you are symptom-free, you may reintroduce the food into the diet. A word of caution: moderation should be used in regard to your allergic foods. Overconsumption of any food can result in food intolerance.

4. Certain foods to which you are severely allergic may need to be avoided forever. This is particularly true if you have significant health problems.

WHY *YOU* SHOULD HAVE A FOOD ALLERGY TEST

The above gives further credence to my belief that, in the case of the chronically ill individual, it is difficult to design a proper diet without knowing what the food allergies are.

I have a wheat allergy. Whenever I eat it, I tire easily. If I have a big enough dose, I fall asleep at my desk. One of my patients knows when I have eaten a piece of bread with lunch. I have an observable loss in my ability to concentrate so much so, that she would say, "You've eaten wheat today." Wheat is really the only food I crave. However, I never made the connection until I had a Food Intolerance Test performed on myself. The only other reliable way to find out would have been to stay away from wheat for a month or two, and then re-introduce it. Most of us are not that disciplined.

I firmly believe you must do just as I did and find out exactly what your allergies are. You have only one chance to live life to its fullest. You deserve the finest health care. Medicine today is geared to give you the best. Don't skimp when it comes to your health.

Fortunately, your doctor, providing he is open-minded and willing to help, can have this test done for you. You do not have to come all the way to my office to have it done. All he needs to do is order a special tube

---

* Any food to which you have had a severe allergic reaction to *must be avoided* regardless of results of allergy testing. Your immune system retains a memory of previous allergic exposures which does not always show up in the test results.

from the lab and draw one tube of blood. It is advised that you fast overnight. The blood can then be shipped from any state in the U.S.A. directly to the lab where the test is performed. Within days you will get the results. Once you know your allergies, you can better apply the principles of this book to eat right, stay healthy and remain young. For ordering information and prices, you or your doctor can contact:

NUTRITIONAL TESTING LABORATORIES
Tower 2 - Suite 404 - 1701 Golf Rd.
Rolling Meadows, Illinois 60008
Phone: (708) 640-1377

Discovering your food allergies is an integral component in the journey towards feeling better, having more energy and living a happier, healthier life. Give yourself that special treat — it will be well worth it!

CHAPTER 10
What Your Allergies Mean

This chapter provides the best results once it is determined what foods you are allergic to. Even so, the information contained herein may be relevant in the endeavor to eat right.

There are several categories of potentially allergic foods and food additives, which include the following:

- Protein-rich foods
- Sugars
- Fruits
- Vegetables
- Grains
- Nuts and seeds
- Spices
- Natural chemicals
- Synthetic chemicals
- Fats and oils

PROTEIN-RICH FOODS

Examples of protein allergy include intolerance to seafood, fish, pork, beef, milk, chicken, cheese and soybeans. Those who are allergic to several proteins may be deficient in certain substances used in the digestion of protein, such as pancreatic enzymes. These enzymes are required before proteins can be completely broken down. Vitamin B-6 and zinc are needed to keep digestive enzymes in an active state. Incompletely digested proteins can be absorbed intact, causing an allergic response. In these instances, immune cells in the blood attack the circulating food proteins as if they are foreign invaders. Allergy to foods rich in protein can result in severe reactions, including asthma attacks, joint pain, hives, swollen throat, and even allergic shock. Such individuals may be sensitive to the actual protein particles or to some other ingredient (such as the iodine in shrimp).

SUGARS

Allergies to sugar include cane and beet sugar, molasses, maple syrup, malt syrup, sorghum, and honey. Most reactions to honey are to the heated and refined varieties.

If an individual has several sugar allergies, it is likely that poor adrenal gland function exists. The adrenal glands help "burn" sugars and starches as a source of fuel. Frequent consumption of highly refined sugars such as cane sugar places great stress upon the adrenal glands.

The immune system reacts to sugar as if it were a poison. Sugar actually depresses immune function. Therefore, sugar sensitivity and allergy is common. It is seen in a variety of conditions including yeast infection, hypoglycemia, diabetes, PMS, obesity, hyperactivity, high blood pressure, heart disease and psychological disorders to name a few.

CASE HISTORY:
Mental confusion, depression and memory loss eliminated.

Mr. F, a 36-year-old male was in distress when he came to see me. He was losing his memory, fighting depression, and had feelings of mental confusion and agitation. When I first saw him, he was nervous and agitated. Upon discussing his condition with him, I discovered that his diet as a child was heavy in refined sugar, and that he currently ate significant amounts of sugar on a daily basis.

A Food Intolerance Test was performed which revealed that Mr. F had severe sugar allergies (white sugar, molasses, and malt syrup). He was placed on a diet very low in sugars and was even restricted in the amount of natural sugar (fruit, bread, etc.) he could consume. Improvement was rapid, with the depression and confusion clearing within 2 weeks. The improvement in memory took a bit longer, and it was restored to normal within 4 months. Today Mr. F is a much happier man, and, due to the improved sense of well being, is pursuing the jobs and goals which he has always desired, proving that *it is not always in your head.* Fortunately, Mr. F sought out this preventive and curative approach before the shrinks got to him. However, there are many who have never had the chance to try nutritional cures for their mental symptoms. Many a case of chronic depression, mood imbalances, psychosis, mania, and anxiety could be cured by a nutritional approach *without the use of mind-altering drugs.* The nutritionally oriented practitioner must take the attitude of finding out *why* these mental symptoms exist, and not just automatically assume they are psychiatric in nature.

CASE HISTORY:
Alzheimer's-like disease with near complete memory loss dramatically improved.

Joe, a pleasant 65-year-old retired painter had one major problem — his memory was shot. In fact, he was an hour and a half late for his first appointment, as he could not remember the directions his wife had given him even though he had her written directions in the car! He was tested for food allergies. Routine blood chemistries were also performed. It was found that he was extremely allergic to sugar. It was also discovered that his blood sugar was abnormally high. Upon further history (elicited from his wife), it was found that his sugar levels had been elevated for years, but that no one had treated him for it. All the while, sugar continued to form a major part of his diet.

Although all this is astonishing, what was even more fascinating was his dramatic improvement. After three weeks on the treatment program of allergy removal, low carbohydrate diet, and nutritional supplements, he was able to drive to the clinic unassisted and without directions. He continues to experience lapses of memory whenever he cheats on his diet or goes without his supplements. The stricter he is in avoiding sugar and his other allergies, the better is his memory.

As discussed in both of these case histories, proper treatment for the mental patient involves a combination of dietary guidance plus the elimination of any allergies. In addition, nutritional supplements help brighten the picture. The following is a rather comprehensive list of natural substances, vitamins, and minerals which have proven helpful in mental disorders:

AMINO ACIDS

gamma aminobutyric acid (GABA)
glutamic acid
taurine
tryptophan

glutamine
phenylalanine
tyrosine

VITAMINS

B-12
folic acid
niacinamide

pantothenic acid
riboflavin
vitamin C

biotin
niacin
para-amino benzoic
  acid
pyridoxine (B-6)
thiamine
vitamin E

MINERALS

calcium
chromium
magnesium
molybdenum
potassium
zinc

chloride
iodine
manganese
natural lithium
sodium

HERBS

cayenne pepper
ginko biloba
onion extract

garlic extract
ginseng
valerian root

OTHER SUBSTANCES

choline
crude liver extract
fish oils (EPA/DHA)
lecithin

chlorella
essential fatty acids
flax seed oil
inositol

HOW NUTRIENTS AFFECT BRAIN CHEMISTRY

There are several mechanisms by which nutrients improve brain function. I have listed below three of the most important ones:

1. **By increasing the production within the brain of natural chemicals known as *neurotransmitters*.**

   Just as the name suggests, these substances help the neurons (brain cells) transmit messages back and forth within the brain. Neurotransmitters also are responsible for sending messages down the spinal cord, which then transmits them to the internal organs. Thus, a deficiency of nutrients within the brain can affect tissues or organs anywhere in the body. Take vitamin B-6, for example. If even a mild deficiency exists — you may remember from Chapter 2 that nearly 7 out of 10 Americans are deficient — a decrease in neurotransmitter synthesis will occur. Without adequate levels of neurotransmitters, the entire nervous system can become disabled. This presents a two-fold problem for the allergy patients. They may develop mental symptoms, plus their defenses for fighting allergic reactions are weakened. The nerves control the function of every organ, tissue, and cell in the body. Even the immune system is controlled by them. Thus, for the long-term treatment of allergies, it is advised that any nutritional deficiencies affecting the brain be identified and corrected. In these cases, diagnostic testing for nutritional deficiency may be necessary.

2. **By improving circulation within the brain**

   Without proper blood flow, the brain cannot get the nutrients it needs. Yes, vitamins and minerals are important to the brain, but even more critical are fuel and oxygen. For fuel, the brain relies on glucose, and oxygen is needed to help burn it into energy. The brain uses 20% of the oxygen produced in the body. Even a mild reduction in blood flow to the brain leads to an oxygen deficit, which then causes symptoms such as memory loss, mental fatigue, and irritability.

Herbs, such as ginko biloba and ginseng increase blood flow to the brain. So do certain vitamins, particularly niacin, vitamin B-6, and vitamin E. You can bet that the function of your nervous system will improve if you take nutrients such as these which improve blood flow to the brain.

3. **By reducing or eliminating the transmission of abnormal nerve signals within the brain.**

In some individuals, the neurons in the brain generate all kinds of garbled, disordered messages. These messages actually build up and clog the brain's ability to send the internal organs appropriate signals. Certain nutrients effectively block the production of the aberrant messages, giving the brain cells time to normalize. They include tryptophan, tyrosine, GABA, glutamine, folic acid, vitamin B-6, niacin, choline, inositol, potassium, and magnesium.

FRUITS

Most everyone knows that citrus fruits are a common cause of allergy. This is true for most citrus fruits, although allergies to grapefruit are somewhat rare. A surprisingly high incidence of lemon and lime allergies are being seen. This may be caused by a reaction to the potent, essential oils contained in the rind of these fruits. In addition, the chemicals and dyes used on them are toxic to the immune system. These chemicals are concentrated mainly in the rinds.

Another category of "allergy fruits" are those which naturally contain salicylates. Salicylates are powerful chemicals in the same family as aspirin. They are found in fairly large amounts in several fruits including apples, apricots, grapes, oranges, blackberries, raspberries, cherries, strawberries, tomatoes, peaches, plums, prunes, nectarines, and currants. Almonds also contain a high amount, and 15 almonds have as much aspirin-like pain killing power as is found in a single aspirin.

Some fruits rarely cause allergy. A partial list includes:

- apricots (despite their salicylate content)
- cantaloupe
- guava
- mango
- pears
- avocado
- figs
- kiwi fruit
- papaya
- watermelon

CASE HISTORY:

Childhood asthma cured in a 9-year-old boy.

Johnny had asthma attacks about once per week, although during the summer the frequency of these attacks decreased somewhat. His mother had tried everything from drugs to dietary changes. When I first saw him, he was taking several asthma medications.

A Food Intolerance Test was performed. When the test results arrived, it was no surprise that he was highly allergic to salicylates, since they have been well established by the medical profession to provoke asthma attacks. Removal of salicylate-containing foods and medicines resulted in a gradual but complete cure of his asthma. In addition, he was told to stay off refined sugar, flour, and oils, and his diet was supplemented with B-complex vitamins and essential fatty acids.

VEGETABLES

Vegetables are certainly as natural as a food can get. Yet, it is possible to develop an allergy to them. Are you, by chance, eating nothing but salads and still not losing weight? An allergy to lettuce or any number of salad vegetables could be the culprit.

CASE HISTORY:

Lettuce allergy causes weight gain.

Mrs. T had a history of a persistent weight problem despite dieting. Among other things, she was found to be allergic to lettuce and endive which she ate daily while dieting. After removing these allergic offenders, she rapidly lost 15 pounds.

THAT CHILD MAY BE SNUBBING HIS NOSE FOR A REASON

There may be good reason why a child refuses to eat certain vegetables such as peas or asparagus. Instinctively, the child may be aware that the food doesn't agree with his system. Forcing the child to eat any allergy-causing foods only makes the allergy worse. In my experience, allergies can be determined more accurately in children ages nine and above. By this time, the immune system has developed enough that the allergies will show up.

Vegetable allergies can be related to conditions under which the vegetables are grown. Celery that is exposed to excess amounts of ultraviolet light may contain toxins known as *furocumarins* which can cause a relatively severe allergic reaction. Alfalfa sprouts contain a potent chemical which can be toxic to the immune system. Corn, especially if stored in elevators, often becomes contaminated with toxins secreted by molds, including aflatoxin. The immune system often reacts violently to contaminated corn or its by-products, such as corn syrup, corn starch, corn oil, dextrin, or corn flour.

Pesticide and herbicide contamination of fresh vegetables is rampant. Unfortunately, most fresh vegetables, unless organically grown, contain residues of these toxic chemicals. Most of the residues are on the outside of the plant. Even so, enough pesticide or herbicide molecules can get into the body to cause an allergic reaction. The best way to solve this is to buy only organically-grown vegetables. However, this is not always feasible, and most supermarkets do not carry organic produce. At the time of this printing, several major supermarket chains have begun carrying a small line of organically grown fruits and vegetables.

Another solution is to soak your vegetables in a compound called *Basic-H*. This completely natural product effectively removes residues of pesticides, herbicides, fertilizers, waxes, and other chemicals found on the outside of the plant. Only a few drops in a bucket of water will do the trick. This procedure will greatly reduce the degree of allergic sensitivity to vegetables, since many vegetable allergies are caused more by contaminants than by the actual food itself. Basic-H can be purchased from a Shaklee distributor, or by mail order:

PHYSICIAN'S HEALTH DESIGN
804 Loretta Dr.
Goodlettsville, Tennessee 37072
(615) 859-7846

Don't worry, though. Fresh vegetables are still an excellent food choice and, overall, contain far less contaminants than do processed or canned ones. It is wise to include as many fresh vegetables in your diet as is possible.

GRAINS

Grain intolerance may well be the most common allergy. Individuals with grain allergies may react to the protein portion of grains. This wheat protein is known as *gluten*. Gluten intolerance can lead to several problems including intestinal inflammation, malabsorption of vitamins and minerals, blood sugar imbalances, and mental disorders. Gluten-containing grains include wheat, rye, buckwheat, barley, oats, and millet. Headaches are commonly caused by grain allergies, as pointed out in this case history.

CASE HISTORY:

Twenty years of migraines cured

Mrs. Z had been plagued with severe migraine headaches which occurred as often as every day. She had a history of headaches for over 20 years. As she was a receptionist in a doctor's office, the headaches often interfered with her work. The quality of her life was reduced significantly due to the pain. She had been all over the country seeking help including the Mayo Clinic and several centers specializing in the treatment of headaches.

Food intolerance testing proved her to be highly allergic to wheat and rye. By removing these foods from her diet and providing the appropriate nutritional support, her headaches were brought under control. Today, Mrs. Z is headache-free. If she cheats and eats anything containing wheat or rye, such as a pancake or a piece of toast, her headaches return.

Four trips to famous medical clinics across the country provided Mrs. Z with little or no help. Yet, it is amazing that results this striking can be achieved simply by removing a few allergic foods from the diet.

WHEAT ALLERGY COULD MEAN A WILD KID

Those who have children deemed to be "hyperactive", please take note. It is likely that the child has allergies, and wheat is one of the top offenders. Wheat affects the brain by two mechanisms. First, it may cause a drop in blood sugar. This is especially true of refined wheat products, such as white flour. Wheat products which are heavily refined contain little or no fiber. Without fiber, the starch from the wheat is rapidly turned into sugar. This causes excess amounts of insulin to be released, leading to a drop in the blood sugar level. When the blood sugar drops, mental symptoms are likely to occur. The brain's only fuel is glucose, and its function is greatly affected when blood glucose levels fall. Second, wheat proteins once entering the bloodstream, can be carried to the brain, where they attach to brain cells at sites called *receptors*. Various types of receptors exist on the cell membranes of brain cells, but most important are those set up to receive insulin. These are the receptors to which the wheat proteins attach! Insulin is needed to drive glucose into brain cells, and, without it, the brain cannot be properly fueled, thus leading to a loss of mental and nerve function. This may be manifested as poor concentration, learning impairment, and/or behavioral disorders. Wheat is double trouble if you are allergic to it.

WHEAT IS EVERYWHERE

It is nearly impossible to buy a packaged, canned, or frozen food from the supermarket without finding within it some wheat or wheat derivative. I would venture to say that at least 70% of all processed foods contain either wheat, wheat flour, breadings, malt, or other unspecified wheat derivatives. Flour is often added by food manufacturers as a thickening agent, although this information is not always listed on the label.

Don't panic if you suspect you are allergic to wheat. There are lots of other foods left such as fruits, vegetables, meats, nuts, and milk products. Always remember to concentrate on what you *can* have, not what you cannot have. This will make life much easier.

NUTS AND SEEDS

Peanuts are the most common nut or seed allergy. Actually, they are not nuts, belonging instead to the legume family. Sensitivity to peanuts often begins in early childhood. Individuals can also be sensitive to walnuts, pecans, cashews, pistachios, sunflower seeds, filberts, and sesame seeds. Nuts, especially walnuts, contain fatty acids which, if rancid, can be toxic to white blood cells. This toxicity can then lead to an allergic response. Symptoms ranging from headaches to a cold or sore throat may result.

SPICES

Spice sensitivity seems to be on the rise. As to the reason why, one can only guess. Most spices are irradiated before they are distributed for sale. Radiation alters the internal chemistry of food, making sensitivity more likely. Mint is a particularly common spice that causes allergy. If you are sensitive to several spices, there may be a weakness in your immune system. Some spices contain chemicals such as alkaloids (found in pepper) or certain rancid oils which can negatively react with the immune system.

NATURAL CHEMICALS

Other chemicals naturally occurring in foods can evoke allergic reactions. It is interesting to note that there are more natural chemicals in existence than synthetic ones. Only a few of these natural chemicals are strong enough to cause allergies. However, many allergic reactions go unnoticed, and a form of tolerance to the causative substance can be developed. This is true with coffee and cocoa. Both of these beans contain a variety of chemicals, although they are best known for their caffeine content. In addition, cocoa contains a substance known as *theobromine*, which can be harmful to the digestive tract and immune system. Coffee itself can be toxic, especially if consumed in excess.

CASE HISTORY:
Coffee causes Irritable Bowel Syndrome

Mrs. G was a 10 to 20 cup a day coffee drinker. She had a history of Irritable Bowel Syndrome. This condition often resulted in mucous and blood in her stool along with severe abdominal pain. After she quit consuming coffee, the irritable bowel attacks subsided. Some years later, she happened to get a job in my office. On occasion, her colon problems would flare up. She was not sure what caused these flare ups, but she did admit to having an occasional cup of coffee. The Food Intolerance Test showed she was extremely sensitive to several natural chemicals including salycilates and coffee. Upon eliminating her occasional cup of coffee, the flare-ups disappeared.

SYNTHETIC CHEMICALS

Today, hundreds of thousands of synthetic chemicals are manufactured by various chemical companies. Over 6,000 different chemicals are now available to be added to our foods. It seems that food manufacturers and processors have an open fist policy. They dump as many chemicals into our foods as they like. There is now a trend, due to consumer demand, to provide additive-free foods. Yet, for many, the damage has already been done. More and more people are becoming allergic to the chemicals in our food. It makes sense. The immune system recognizes the chemical as being foreign and, therefore, attacks it. A biochemical reaction then occurs between the toxic chemical and the immune system. The result is symptoms ranging from flu-like sensations to headaches. Eventually, exposure to the chemical will automatically result in an allergic response. Some of the more common chemicals that can be tested include saccharin, Nutra Sweet, MSG, sulfites, pesticides, and herbicides.

FATS AND OILS

A food allergy or intolerance can occur to animal and/or vegetable fats. Both can be equally bad. Butter allergy is common. This is due in part to the chemicals put in butter, especially *Butter Yellow*, a hydrocarbon made from coal tar. Allergies to olive, safflower, corn, sunflower, and cottonseed oil can also develop. Most margarine is made with corn and/or cottonseed oil. If you are allergic to either of these, this would be another good reason to avoid margarine. As a rule, if you are allergic to a food, you will also need to avoid the oils that are made from that food. For example, an olive allergy means that olive oil needs to be avoided.

CASE HISTORY:

A 33-year-old male (Mr. C) was plagued with chronic nasal drainage. His nose became easily congested, and he often developed sneezing spells. At times, his nose would run so profusely that he had to leave his place of work due to the embarrassment. He also noticed an increased vulnerability to colds and flu.

Testing showed that he had the maximum reaction to butter. Whenever he ate large amounts of it, he noticed an increase in nasal discharge. Apparently, the Butter Yellow dye caused a depression of his immune system, since both his allergy symptoms and immune function improved dramatically when he avoided butter. Removal of butter alone led to a 90% improvement in his symptoms.

THE ROLE OF THE ADRENAL GLANDS

People who have numerous allergies (to me, numerous means 30 or more of a possible 205), have weakened adrenal glands. The adrenal glands are the most important organ for fighting allergies. They produce hormones such as cortisone which help prevent allergic reactions and/or decrease their intensity. The adrenals can be strengthened with the appropriate type and dosage of nutrients. Stress reduction and removal of the offending foods are also important. Eating excessive quantities of sugars and starches weaken the adrenal glands. This is one more reason why the reduced carbohydrate diet described in this book is so beneficial. Adrenal-enhancing nutrients help by improving symptoms related to existing allergies and by reducing the tendency to develop further allergies. These nutrients include:

- vitamin A (helps in the synthesis of adrenal cells)
- vitamin C (prevents the breakdown of adrenal hormones and aids in hormone synthesis)
- pantothenic acid (invaluable in preventing damage to the adrenal glands; it is required for the synthesis of adrenal hormones)
- vitamin B-6
- thiamine
- sodium (needed to help the adrenals maintain fluid and electrolyte balance)
- magnesium
- manganese
- potassium
- selenium (prevents the adrenals from being damaged or infected)
- vitamin E
- bioflavonoids (helps prevent the adrenal cells from degenerating)

Many allergic patients actually have a deficiency in sodium. Often, such individuals crave salt. The reason is that the weakened adrenal glands can no longer produce enough of the hormone which causes the kidneys to retain salt. This hormone is known as *aldosterone*. Thus, without sufficient aldosterone, salt is lost into the urine. In such patients, food should be cooked with salt, and a heavy hand should be used with the salt shaker.* In addition, snacks that are salty are advisable.

ALLERGIES AND INTESTINAL MALABSORPTION

Food allergies cause a reaction which leads to inflammation in the intestinal wall. Excess quantities of mucous are formed by cells lining the intestine to soften the blow. This inflammation, along with the excess mucous, promotes a malabsorption of vitamins, minerals, and other nutrients. Wheat allergy is often associated with zinc malabsorption. Multiple grain allergies, known medically as *gluten intolerance*, cause a malabsorption of virtually all the vitamins and minerals. Allergy to milk or milk products can cause malabsorption of most all the minerals and many vitamins as well.

A simple way you can remedy this is to take the **Intestinal Rebuilder Cocktail**. Just add one packet of chlorella granules to 6 ounces of aloe vera juice. A special type of aloe vera juice is now available which is approximately three times more effective than any other on the market (see appendix B). This aloe vera juice helps soothe and heal the wounded intestinal lining. This is due in part to its rich content of *mucopolysac-charides*, substances which are critical to maintaining a healthy intestinal wall. Chlorella also helps heal, and with its rich content of nucleic acids (RNA and DNA), it assists the growth of new cells throughout the entire gastrointestinal tract.

I'll bet you are wondering what your allergy profile is. When you find out what your allergies are, this chapter will serve as your guide.

* Pure sea salt is the best type to use, since commercial salt contains aluminum and sugar. The aluminum is added as an anti-caking agent.

CHAPTER 11
Alcoholism: The Number 3 Killer?

Alcoholism is a problem on the rise. Despite current approaches to treatment, the incidence of this disease continues to climb. An interesting statistic is that over 25,000 new alcoholics crop up each year in New York state alone. In the United States today, there are some 15 to 20 million alcoholics. That is almost one out of every ten people. This being the case, it should not be a surprise that approximately 50 billion dollars are spent each year in relation to the physical, mental and social repercussions of this rampant disease.

Alcoholism may well be the number three killer. It is unique in that death can be caused by a variety of mechanisms — it can kill both the alcoholic and victimize the innocent. It causes or contributes to the death of over 100,000 people annually. Statistics show that the major factor in fatal industrial accidents is imbibing on the job. A much greater concern is that nearly one out of every two deaths from car accidents is alcohol-related. Also, a high percentage of mass transportation accidents, including airline mishaps, are related to the drinking habits of the crew.

A second way alcohol can kill is through its direct effect upon the human body. Alcoholics suffer fatalities from both the number one and number two killers, heart disease and cancer. In addition, long-term alcohol consumption brings on its own brand of fatal disease: cirrhosis of the liver.

The current approach to treating the alcoholic has been ineffective. Yet, it is interesting that alcoholism is the only major disease for which physicians refer care to the lay public. The standard approach has been drug detoxification, counseling, and group therapy. Extensive education programs both for the alcoholic and his/her family members are also applied. Unfortunately, results are poor. Less than 15% of alcoholics are cured. Therefore, it is important to use *any* method possible to resolve this problem. For reasons beyond comprehension, the nutritional and dietary basis of this condition have been totally neglected by the medical establishment. Yet, poor nutrition has as much to do with the development of alcoholism as it does with any other disease.

Nutritional factors contributing to the cause of alcoholism were studied extensively in the 1940's. The lid of the nutrition/alcoholism coffin has only recently been re-opened. The life of many an alcoholic who *wishes to be helped* can be saved by the principles discussed in this chapter. I will review some of the current scientific facts indicating the tremendous havoc which alcohol causes in respect to the body's nutritional status and give you some pearls of wisdom on how to most effectively treat this dreadful disease.

WHAT IS ALCOHOL?

Alcohol is nearly 100% carbohydrate. It originates primarily from starches which are highly refined and fermented. It is, at best, a fuel devoid of essential nutrients. Alcohol provides calories which, according to the researcher, Lieber, are "empty."

Most alcoholic beverages are derived from grains which were originally nutritious. To make alcohol, brewers and distillers remove the germ and outer coatings (bran) of these grains, using only the starchy portion. This constitutes a loss of nearly all the fat soluble vitamins which are located in the fatty germ, and most of the B-vitamins, which are found both in the germ and the bran. Hard liquor, being distilled, is entirely free of nutrients. The minerals, vitamins, and trace elements from raw materials such as corn mash, rye, or barley, are left behind in the residues. These are discarded, or used as a nutritious feed supplement for cattle.

Even worse are beverages such as brandy, rum, and liqueurs, which are made from distilled alcohol *plus added sugar*. Refined sugar itself is 99.9% nutrient free. Often, when individuals mix drinks such as cocktails, they actually add sugar to what is already nothing but pure, nutrient-free carbohydrate.

Thus it is accurate to say that alcoholic beverages are essentially protein, fat, vitamin, and mineral free. Contrary to popular belief, beer is little better. Most beer is made from the starchy part of barley. It is much lower in B-vitamins than some are led to believe. Beer, with its diuretic effect, purges from the body more vitamins and minerals than it provides. What little nutrition it does have comes from the yeast it contains which is added during the fermentation process.

Wine also contains a minimal amount of nutrients. Red wine is a bit more nutritious, being a product from fermented fruits. Only the juices from the fruits are used. Thus, most of the original nutrients are left behind in the skins and pulp. However, some wines are high in iron, especially red wines. As discussed in Chapters 7 and 8, this extra iron may do more harm than good.

ADDICTIVE ACTIONS

The highly refined nature of alcohol accounts for much of its addictive power. This also accounts for its drug-like action on human chemistry and behavior. It should be noted that the same is true of narcotic drugs which are also of plant origin. They too are highly refined in order to make them more potent. It is a general rule that the more refined a narcotic is, the more powerful its addictive nature. Crack is an example, since it is even more refined than cocaine. The same is true of alcohol. In all sense of the word, alcohol is not a food. It is a drug and in the body it acts like a drug. Thus, the various organs of the body, rather than being nourished by alcohol, are "affected" by it. Alcohol can be defined as a food-derived chemical with addictive and drug-like action.

HOW ALCOHOLISM DEVELOPS

Most alcoholics develop their disease gradually. Some people, especially teenagers, become alcoholics literally overnight. In most cases, there is a profound craving for alcoholic beverages, and for that matter, sugars and starches. These cravings indicate the existence of an imbalance in body chemistry. This makes a person just that much more vulnerable to developing the addiction.

ARE YOU GENETICALLY SUSCEPTIBLE?

It is now generally believed that those who have a significant family history of alcoholism are more vulnerable to the disease. The alcoholic gene, as it is often called, seems to involve a craving for alcohol and other refined carbohydrates, such as sugar. The more deficient in nutrients individuals with this gene become, the more likely they are to crave alcohol as a stimulant. They may seek alcohol for the temporary high that it gives.

SOCIAL DRINKING — THE BEGINNINGS OF ALCOHOLISM?

Many alcoholics fall pray to the typical social drinking norms. Advertising by the alcohol industry would have us believe that consuming its beverages is synonymous with having a "good time." Others feel pressured by peers to begin drinking. Today, even children in grade school are feeling this strain.

Much alcoholism has its origin in colleges, where there is intense pressure to party and have a good time through the use of stimulants. Often, combined with a diet high in sugar and starch (the typical college diet has 50-70% of its calories as carbohydrates), the stage for long-term addiction is set.

Once an individual becomes an alcoholic, he begins to gradually replace food calories with alcoholic ones. As the disease develops, he shows a greater aversion to food, particularly wholesome food. Alcohol eventually crowds food out and can account for up to 80% of an alcoholic's caloric intake.

HOW ALCOHOL AFFECTS THE BODY

Alcohol is a simple molecule. Once it enters the stomach and intestines, it is absorbed rapidly. The presence of food in the stomach slows its absorption. Within one to two hours, nearly all the ingested alcohol gets into the system. Once in the blood, most alcohol is taken up by the liver, which attempts to break it down. The rest is excreted unchanged by the lungs (in the breath), the kidneys (in the urine), and through the skin.

Some liver damage can occur even from as few as two or three drinks per week. This condition is known as fatty liver. You may be wondering how this could occur. The liver is the only organ containing large quantities of the enzyme (known medically as *alcohol dehydrogenase*) which can metabolize alcohol. Thus, it bears the brunt of the damage.

NIACIN DEFICIENCY AND ALCOHOLISM

In the liver, alcohol is broken down for purposes of becoming a fuel, since the body can find no other useful function for it. These reactions lead to the formation of a potent chemical known as *acetaldehyde*. The liver attempts to detoxify this chemical through a reaction which requires niacin (vitamin B-3). If there is a deficiency of niacin, even more of this chemical accumulates. The result is damage to the liver cells. Once damaged, the liver cells cannot metabolize alcohol or other sugars adequately and the cells become infiltrated with fat. Eventually, the cells become scarred and no longer function adequately. This is cirrhosis of the liver.

You may recall from Chapter 2 that most Americans are deficient in niacin. The alcoholic is even more likely to have a major niacin deficiency.

DIRECT TOXIC EFFECTS

In addition, alcohol itself is directly toxic to cells and cell membranes. The cell membrane's fatty-acid coating is disrupted by the alcohol molecules. Direct damage can also occur to the stomach and intestinal wall as well as to the brain and spinal cord. The pancreas is also damaged by alcohol, and it is no surprise that alcoholics are much more likely to develop hypoglycemia, diabetes, or even pancreatic cancer.

HYPOGLYCEMIA — THE ALCOHOLIC'S CURSE

Hypoglycemia is a major problem in promoting the alcohol addiction. When blood sugar levels drop, the alcoholic becomes nervous and/or agitated and seeks to correct this by having a drink. Blood sugar imbalances can lead to violence, mood swings, and erratic behavior. Normally, blood sugar levels are lowest in the a.m. Thus, for the alcoholic, the morning can be a horrible time, since blood sugar levels are at their lowest. This can also be a difficult time for close family members who have to deal with the alcoholic's mood swings, depression, and potential violence. Alcoholics also experience blood sugar drops during periods of psychological or emotional stress and are then more vulnerable to having drinking binges. Even mild exercise can lead to a significant drop in their blood sugar levels. This is how delicate the blood sugar mechanism is in most alcoholics. This fact must be clearly understood in order to appreciate the treatment I suggest — that ALCOHOLICS CANNOT HANDLE REFINED SUGARS OR STARCHES IN ANY FORM. In fact, they may not even be able to handle natural sources of sugar or starch, such as an orange or baked potato, without having blood sugar fits.

THE RIGHT ALCOHOLIC DIET

We talked briefly about the wrong alcoholic diet, i.e., one high in alcohol, sugar and starch. The right diet is rich in protein, fresh vegetables, nuts, seeds, and some fruits. The best diet is one in which grains are omitted entirely. Why? Because most alcoholics are allergic to grains. I recommend that each alcoholic have a Food Intolerance Test, since these and other allergies may play a role in the maintenance of the disease, as is demonstrated by the following case histories:

CASE HISTORY: Weekend beer binger kicks the habit.

Mr. E, an aspiring building contractor, had a problem. After a week of hard work he celebrated the weekend by drinking a beer. The problem was that once he started drinking he couldn't stop. He would chug up to twenty beers at a sitting. This, by definition, qualifies him as an alcoholic.

On the insistence of his wife, he came to my clinic for testing. It was found that he was allergic to barley and Brewer's yeast, the two major ingredients of beer! In addition, he was very sensitive to cane sugar, molasses, and rye, all of which are used to make alcohol. By removing these allergic foods, Mr. E has been able to control his drinking binges entirely. His home is a happier place, and he and his wife are now the proud parents of their first child.

CASE HISTORY: Chronic alcoholic in DTs successfully detoxified

When I first saw Mr. McD, he was in obvious distress. He was as pale as a ghost, and what I noticed most was that he was trembling. His hands and arms were shaking so much that he was even making me nervous. Anyone who lives with a chronic alcoholic knows that this is a sign of delirium tremens (DTs), which means that the alcoholic is in serious trouble and that his life could be in danger.

The normal treatment for DTs is, of course, drugs. These drugs are used to suppress the nervous agitation, tremors, and any potentially violent behavior. Yet, the drugs do nothing to treat the primary cause of the DTs: *nutritional deficiency.*

DTs are nothing more than a manifestation of end-stage damage to the nervous system resulting from severe vitamin-mineral deficiencies, alcohol induced, of course. The nutrients most involved are thiamine, vitamin B-6, niacin, vitamin B-12, vitamin C, magnesium, and selenium. This was the basis for the treatment administered to Mr. McD. He too had allergies, with positive reactions to Brewer's yeast and malt. Without the use of drugs, Mr. McD's tremors were successfully eliminated, and within two weeks he was completely off alcohol. He hasn't had a drink since, and this was without AA meetings or support groups. Just nutrition and positive, firm advice from the doctor were used — that was Mr. McD's formula for a cure.

A wide range of food allergies occur in alcoholics and, to a degree, these allergies are responsible for their addictive behavior. For this reason, it is difficult to design a proper diet without knowing what the allergies are. However, the following are some general guidelines that can be helpful:

1.   Avoid all grains and grain derivatives. This includes whole grains.

2.   Eliminate sugars, molasses, malt, maple syrup, and other sweeteners from the diet.

3.   Control the hypoglycemia by eating a high-protein breakfast and at least two between-meal snacks per day. Follow the diet and recipes contained in this book, adding snacks between meals of nuts, seeds, sliced vegetables, and meats.

4.   Throw all your booze, beer and wine away.*

There is one grain derivative I do recommend: rice bran. Rice bran is the substance left over when brown rice is refined into white rice. It was formerly known as "rice polishings." You are probably unaware that alcoholism is in essence a form of beriberi, and rice polishings were the remedy first used to cure this disease. Rice bran can still be used to cure, and can truly help the alcoholic recover from his/her disease.**

Why is rice bran so effective? Because it is one of the richest natural sources of thiamine (vitamin B-1), niacin (vitamin B-3), and magnesium, which are the three major nutritional deficiencies seen in the alcoholic. The recommended dose is two tablespoons of rice bran three times per day added to juice or over food. In stubborn cases, try taking two heaping tablespoons every four hours. Rice bran is also rich in chromium, a mineral critical for maintaining proper blood sugar levels.

DEFICIENCIES GALORE

Alcoholics develop a wide range of nutritional deficiencies. In addition to vitamins and minerals, they become deficient in essential fatty acids and proteins. No surprise then, that the structural changes in an alcoholic's liver mimic those seen in a starvation victim. The following is a partial list of the nutrients which are deficient in most alcoholics:

1. vitamin A
2. vitamin C (the number one cause of scurvy in alcoholism)
3. vitamin E
4. vitamin D
5. vitamin K
6. vitamin B-1
7. vitamin B-2
8. vitamin B-3
9. vitamin B-5
10. vitamin B-6
11. biotin
12. vitamin B-12
13. folic acid
14. essential fatty acids
15. amino acids and proteins
16. enzymes
17. zinc
18. cobalt
19. selenium
20. calcium
21. phosphorus
22. magnesium
23. manganese
24. potassium
25. chromium

*No long-term alcoholic should go "cold turkey" unless under the care of a physician or reputable treatment institution.

** An excellent source of rice bran is made by Pacific Rice under the brand name *Vita Fiber* (see appendix B).

As you can see, there is hardly a single known nutrient that is not deficient. Some nutrients, however, are more important than others, as described below.

NUTRIENTS FOR DECREASING ALCOHOLIC CRAVINGS

Harrison's Textbook of Medicine states that most alcoholics are deficient in protein. No wonder. They are simply not getting enough in their diets. In addition, alcohol interferes with the absorption of amino acids, the building blocks which make up proteins.

Dr. Roger Williams aptly described how glutamine, an amino acid found in high-protein foods such as eggs, milk, and meat has a protective effect against the cravings for alcohol. Glutamine was first studied in rats which were given alcohol to drink. These rats eventually craved alcohol so much that they preferred it over water. The administration of glutamine wiped out these cravings, and the rats returned to drinking water. With humans, similar decreases in cravings have been seen, although doses as high as 3 to 4 grams of glutamine per day may be necessary. Another nutrient proven to decrease cravings is the fatty acid found in evening primrose oil. This natural oil is called *gamma-linolenic acid* (GLA). It has been effective in minimizing alcoholic withdrawal symptoms, and helps heal alcohol-induced damage to brain tissue, restoring memory, proper thinking, and reaction time.

B-VITAMINS TO THE RESCUE

Undoubtedly, the most crucial nutrients for detoxifying, curing, or healing the alcoholic are the B-vitamins. Niacin alone has been shown to be curative by some physicians and researchers. Most alcoholics have a severe niacin deficiency. Normally, some niacin can be manufactured from the amino acid tryptophan. The bowel contains bacteria which synthesize niacin. However, long-term alcohol consumption leads to a tryptophan deficiency and causes the destruction of the helpful bowel bacteria. Alcohol destroys niacin in many ways, and this may explain why alcoholics respond so well to it. Dr. Robert Smith has noted a 50-60% success using niacin alone in curing alcoholic priests. Over half of some 500 priests enjoy freedom from alcoholism five years after the initial treatment with niacin. No doubt, niacin helps detoxify alcoholics and makes it easier for them to overcome the addiction.

For niacin to work over the long haul, it must be taken daily. The brain and other organs of an alcoholic on autopsy show signs of pellagra, the original disease caused by niacin deficiency. Such a critical situation demands that the alcoholic take an adequate dose of niacin daily for life. In addition, foods rich in niacin are highly recommended, particularly rice bran, although calf's liver, chicken, fish, peanuts, and sunflower seeds are also excellent sources.

Niacin's beneficial effects upon the alcoholic are wide in scope. Enriching the diet with niacin-rich foods as well as taking niacin supplements can help prevent the alcoholic from dying young.

THIAMINE — THE MORAL VITAMIN

Thiamine is also universely deficient in the alcoholic. Alcohol destroys thiamine. In addition, the typical diet followed by the alcoholic is low in thiamine. Alcoholics should add thiamine-rich foods to their diet. A fine source of natural thiamine is rice bran. Other good sources include sunflower seeds, pine nuts, wheat germ, soybeans, peanuts, and sesame seeds. These and other foods naturally rich in thiamine are not normal constituents of the alcoholic's diet.

Alcoholics usually develop symptoms secondary to thiamine deficiency. These symptoms include depression, mood swings, hypoglycemia, insomnia, muscle weakness, indigestion, nerve pains, nausea, and nervousness. Later, as the deficiency becomes more profound, alcoholics may develop a degenerative disease of the brain or spinal cord. Thiamine is needed for the proper function of both of these organs. In fact, the function of all nerves in the body is dependent upon thiamine. The finest thiamine supplement I know of is *Allithiamine*. Allithiamine is better tolerated and absorbed than most other thiamine products. For ordering information, contact:

CARDIOVASCULAR RESEARCH
1061-B Shary Circle
Concord, CA 94518
Ph. (415) 827-2636

B-12 AND FOLIC ACID

Vitamin B-12 and folic acid go hand in hand. Alcohol washes both of these vitamins out of the liver, where they are normally stored. When levels of these two vitamins become low enough, the alcoholic develops a form of anemia. With this type of anemia there are enough red cells, but the size and shape of these cells (and, therefore, their function) becomes abnormal. This is known medically as *macrocytic* or *pernicious* anemia. In addition, alcohol, while in the intestines, blocks the absorption of folic acid and B-12.

To restore the proper levels of folic acid, it is recommended that the alcoholic consume large quantities of fresh, green, leafy vegetables. Meats are also a good source. There are only a few good dietary sources of B-12. This is why I would recommend that the alcoholic consume chlorella, preferably Sun Chlorella, which has a form of B-12 that is easily absorbed. The usual dose would be 15 tablets three times daily. However, be careful to start on any new supplement slowly. Alcoholics are usually so full of toxins and poisons that introducing nutrition-rich supplements such as chlorella will cause a temporary detoxification reaction. If an individual starts slowly and works up to the suggested dose, no such reaction should occur. Other food sources of B-12 include red meats, beef liver, clams, fish, crab, eggs, and cheese. In addition, injections of B-12 and folic acid would be valuable. If you are an alcoholic, your doctor may be willing to give you these. I usually recommend that the alcoholic get at least two shots a week for the first month, tapering off to a shot at least once per month as a maintenance.

MINERALS ARE IMPORTANT

Alcohol interferes with the absorption of several minerals. It also leads to the loss of minerals in the urine. Alcoholics lose lots of magnesium in their urine. Magnesium deficiency predisposes alcoholics to sudden death from heart attack or stroke. Magnesium supplements are important, but foods rich in magnesium should be added to the diet. These include rice bran, green leafy vegetables, apricots, figs, chick peas, wheat germ, peanuts, nuts of all types, and spices. Magnesium imparts to certain spices their hot flavor. Magnesium-rich spices include coriander leaf, cayenne pepper, dill weed, celery seed, sage, and mustard. Use lots of spices in your cooking. You might be surprised at the results.

ZINC MAY BE THE MISSING LINK

Nearly every alcoholic has a profound zinc deficiency. Zinc controls many functions which, when disrupted, predispose individuals to alcoholism. It is my contention that zinc deficiency causes certain individuals to become alcoholics. Without adequate zinc, the ability to taste or smell food is compromised. Therefore, the normal appetite for eating wholesome foods is disturbed. Zinc is also needed for the digestion of proteins and for the proper metabolism of essential fatty acids. Zinc deficiency leads to the craving of foods rich in carbohydrates and low in protein and other nutrients, such as alcohol and sugar. The zinc deficient individual often avoids healthy foods which are rich in nutrients, aroma and taste. It has been shown that supplementing the diet with zinc gradually restores these functions to normal and decreases the abnormal cravings for alcohol and sugar.

Alcoholics lose up to 8 times more zinc in their urine than do normal individuals. The ability of the body to absorb and transport zinc is diminished through the toxic effects of alcohol upon the liver. In addition, zinc is required by the liver before alcohol can be metabolized into less toxic substances.

Without zinc, the alcoholic cannot make proper use of other nutrients such as fatty acids, vitamin B-6, and vitamin A. The scope of symptoms related to zinc deficiency include anorexia, hair loss, mental disturbances, depression, anxiety, agitation dry skin, fatigue, impotence, susceptibility to colds or flu, and poor wound healing.

SUMMARY

Alcohol is a poison. It is toxic to tissues and organs throughout the body. It can damage the liver, brain, heart, stomach and intestines. If used in excess, it predisposes to heart disease, sudden death, and cancer. It has been directly related to the cause of cancer of the esophagus, throat, stomach and colon. Alcohol creates its own disease, cirrhosis of the liver. If you avoid alcohol, it may lower the opinion some of your peers or associates have of you. But by doing so, you may well save your life. By the way, in case you are not aware, few people are looked down upon more than the drunkard. By kicking the drinking habit, you'll earn the love and respect of the people who count — your family, friends, and business associates who care about your health and happiness.

CHAPTER 12
Fats Are Not The Killer

Fatty foods are good for you. That's right, it's safe to eat fats. What I really mean is that many foods *naturally high* in fats are healthy to eat. This is the exact opposite of all you have been taught or told. I know that the media and medical profession have got you running scared. People are afraid to even look at foods naturally rich in fats such as eggs, cream, butter, meats, avocados, etc. This is just pure nonsense. Eggs, meats, butter, and other foods naturally rich in fats are some of the most wholesome foods available. On this diet, it is possible to eat as much naturally fat-rich foods as you desire. In fact, you need to get as many natural fats into your diet as possible. As I described in Chapter 5, there is a tremendous need for adding healthy fats into the diet due to the rampant use of poor-quality fats. You may recall from the first chapter that 100% of us are deficient in essential fatty acids. Therefore, it would be wise to eat as much natural fat as possible *on a daily basis*.

A word of caution: it is safe only to eat natural fats. I call these the *good fats*. Some fats are dangerous, and these are the *bad fats*.

Bad fats should be avoided at all costs. These fats have little or no nutritional value. Here is a list of fatty foods and fat sources you must avoid:

- Margarine
- Lard
- Hot dogs
- Processed cheeses (Cheez Whiz, Velveeta, American)
- Deep fried foods
- Vegetable oils (which are not cold-pressed)

- Sausage
- Bratwurst
- Pork rinds
- Bologna
- Mayonnaise

- Salad dressing

- Crisco
- Shortening
- Peanut butter with added hydrogenated fats
- Potato chips or other fried snacks
- Tropical oils (palm kernel, coconut, and cottonseed)
- Baked goods

There are a number of reasons why these particular fats are bad for you. They disrupt digestion by irritating the liver and gallbladder. Like glue, they can stick to the inside of the arteries leading to diseases of the heart and/or arteries. Bad fats weaken the immune system and disrupt the function of the white blood cells. The consumption of some of these fats is associated with an increased risk for cancer.

Recently, the food processing industry has added another vegetable oil to the marketplace — Canola oil. This is made from a plant seed known as rapeseed. While touting the oil for its high content of mono and polyunsaturated fats, they have neglected one fact: Canola oil contains the highly toxic *erucic acid*. Erucic acid is *unfit for human consumption*. For this reason I do not recommend the use of Canola oil. Good fats, on the other hand, are those found naturally within certain wholesome foods. A list includes:

Almonds
Avocado
Beef
Brazil nuts
Butter
Cheese (hard and feta cheeses)
Cottage Cheese
Chicken (with skin)
Duck
Eggs
Filberts
Goat's milk (whole)
Goose
Hazelnuts
Lamb

Macadamia nuts
Olives
Organ meats
Peanuts (roasted)
Peanut butter
Pecans
Pine nuts
Pistachios
Pumpkin seeds
Rice germ
Sesame seeds
Sunflower seeds
Walnuts
Wheat germ
Yogurt (from whole milk)

Believe me, you can eat as much of these foods as you want in terms of the fat content, *without worry*. This is providing that you are not allergic to any of them. These foods are healthier in that, pound for pound, they contain more nutrients than do breads, pasta, rice, oats, and other starchy foods. Plus, they are far more nutritious than the worthless snack foods that almost everyone eats without the least bit of concern. These nutrient-poor snacks include cookies, pastries, chips, candy,

French fries, pizza, and soft drinks. In addition, the fats found in the "good fat" foods actually protect you against heart disease, arthritis, cancer, and many other degenerative diseases.

Would you like to have more energy? Then eat lots of the good fats. Fats are the most efficient energy source. The best example of this I have seen is the national champion college wrestling team — the Iowa Hawkeyes. I observed their dietary habits first hand, since at that time (1976), I was a college wrestler at the University of Northern Iowa which is one of their competitors. Due to the standards in sports nutrition at that time, our team had been instructed to eat *only carbohydrates* before the match. While my team was eating pancakes covered with sugary syrup, to my amazement, the Iowa Hawkeye team members were eating steak and eggs! During that period, the Hawkeyes were the strongest, most powerful college wrestling team ever known. In retrospect, I feel much of their extra edge was due to their ignorance of the sports nutrition "party line" at the time — that pre-game meals should be high in sugar and starch and low in fat.

You too can achieve some of these same benefits — more energy, and if you are an athlete, increased strength and endurance — by eating foods naturally rich in fats. In fact, if more athletes took advantage of these concepts and applied them in their routines, their performance would soar dramatically.

There are many reasons why fats are an excellent source of energy. They are well absorbed and easily utilized as fuel. Fats contain double the caloric energy of proteins or carbohydrates.

MITOCHONDRIA: CELLULAR POWERPLANTS

Within the cells of the human body exist tiny factory-like organs known as *mitochondria*. Mitochondria are responsible for over 90% of the energy production within the cells. These microscopic organs efficiently use fats as a source of energy. In fact, they prefer fat over carbohydrate as an energy source.

You can actually have more energy from eating foods rich in fats than from carbohydrate or sugar-rich foods. Try this for yourself. Tomorrow, eat a breakfast high in carbohydrates, such as cereal with milk and orange juice. The next day, eat a high-fat and protein breakfast, such as three eggs cooked in olive oil or butter with a hamburger patty. Compare how you feel. If you experience an energy let-down between 10:00 a.m. and 2:00 p.m. on the first day, and felt fine on the second, you'll understand my point. Fats sustain your energy longer by providing more cellular energy per pound and by preventing blood sugar swings. In contrast, fluctuations in blood sugar levels are commonly caused by carbohydrate-rich foods.

The good fats and fat-rich foods previously listed are important food sources. They are of particular value for people with the following diseases:

- Cholesterol Elevation
- Hardening of the Arteries
- Hypoglycemia
- Triglyceride Elevation
- Diabetes
- Heart Disease
- Obesity

These are precisely the diseases for which fats have been prohibited! Contrary to popular belief, these diseases respond better to fat-rich foods than to carbohydrates. A good example of this is the recent scientific survey comparing the health aspects of high fat milk products versus skim milk products. A team of eight researchers in Massachusetts found that low fat milk products such as skim milk, yogurt, and cottage cheese increase the risk of cancer. It seems that the milk sugar, galactose, is the culprit rather than the fat.

The complex carbohydrate diet, highly touted by nutritionists across the country, is usually a poor choice for people who have these diseases. A high *natural* fat diet, enriched with lots of vegetables and certain fruits is the preferred choice. The following case history illustrates how this works.

CASE HISTORY:
Corporate executive loses 30 pounds and drops over 90 points on his cholesterol.

Mr. C is a top executive at a major insurance company. His primary concern was that he had a long-term problem with elevated cholesterol. In addition, over a ten year period, he had put on an extra 30 pounds. The extra weight looked disfiguring since Mr. C is a tall man with a medium bone structure, and all that fat went right to his waist. His memory was also failing, and he was plagued particularly with problems in short-term recall. There was some concern that this would have a negative impact on his work.

Previously, Mr. C tried the standard low-fat, low-cholesterol diet, cutting out all foods containing fat such as eggs, cheese, meats, avocados, nuts, etc. While his weight did drop by 15 pounds, his cholesterol stayed the same! Previously, his diet consisted primarily of beans and pasta, with some fruits and vegetables eaten occasionally.

Mr. C was placed on the high healthy fat diet as outlined in Chapter 13. He was told to omit all refined sugars and starches as well as alcoholic beverages from his diet. The results were spectacular. Within 3 months his cholesterol dropped nearly 100 points, and he lost 30 pounds. This was without any exercise. His memory also improved, and he notes that it is better than it has been in years.

How could such a dramatic improvement in weight loss, cholesterol, and circulation (better memory) occur? In Mr. C's case, it was because his body was able to metabolize healthy fats better than carbohydrates, whether they were healthy ones or not.*

There is another factor — remember Chapter 5 — how all those processed foods were laced with refined vegetable oils and hydrogenated fats? These fats mess-up the metabolic machinery. They interfere with thyroid function, and this is the master gland of metabolism. They distort the structure and chemistry of cells within the liver, leading in many cases to elevations in cholesterol, despite their being advertised as causing its reduction. The diet outlined in this book eliminates all foods containing these fats and replaces them with large amounts of essential fats, fats which help normalize the metabolism.

It has even been shown that the essential fats help drive the bad fats right out of the cells. In Mr. C's case, this is precisely what happened, and explains the dramatic improvement in metabolism he experienced.

Now Mr. C can eat natural sugars and starches without automatically putting on weight. Even so, he is advised to stay on the fat-rich diet for the long term. He has more energy, better memory, and improved weight control.

In Chapter 13, you will be given two sample weeks of this diet. If you follow this program, 60 to 70% of your food calories will probably come from fats. However, there is no need for concern. In fact, if your diet consists mostly of processed foods, you are getting that much fat in the diet anyway. The following chart illustrates how this can happen:

PROCESSED FOODS   % OF CALORIES FROM FAT**

Italian dressing	96
Cream cheese	92
Thousand island dressing	90
French dressing	87
Imitation sour cream	86
Sausage	82
Hot dog	81
Bologna	81
Bratwurst	81
Liverwurst	78

* Examples of natural, healthy carbohydrates are brown rice, whole wheat products, potatoes, corn, beans, peas, apples, orange juice, etc.

** These percentages may vary slightly depending upon the method of cooking and/or preparation.

PROCESSED FOODS   % OF CALORIES FROM FAT

American cheese...77
Cole slaw 73
Chocolate covered almonds...............................70
Potato chips, Pringles type 69
Cheese spread...68
Coffee creamer, non-dairy 67
Chicken nuggets...65
Chocolate-covered candy bar with peanuts 64
Frozen egg substitute (made with hydrogenated oils)............64
Potato chips, regular type 62
Brownies..60
Potato salad 59
Corn chips 57
Chocolate kisses..58
Chicken thigh, deep fried...............................58
Wheat thins 56
Cheese puffs 56
Beef tacos 53
Chocolate eclair 53
Cheese and sausage pizza................................52
Doughnut, raised type 51
French fries, deep fried 51
Vanilla ice cream 50
Danish pastry...50
Fish sandwich (with cheese, tartar sauce, and fries) 50
Double burger (with sauce and fries) 50
Tortilla chips 49
Coconut custard pie.....................................48
Macaroni and cheese 48
Pumpkin pie...48
Doughnut, plain, cake type 44
Peanut butter cookie 42
Waffle, plain...36

NATURAL FOODS (AND SPICES)	% OF CALORIES FROM FAT
Butter	100
Olives	95
Pecans	88
Macadamia nuts	93
Coconuts	87
Avocados	88
Walnuts	88
T-bone, broiled	82
Almonds	76
Pistachios	77
Peanuts	71
Poppy seeds	75
Sunflower seeds	76
Pumpkin seeds	76
Pine nuts	75
Lamp chop	74
Feta cheese	73
Hamburger patty, cooked	64
Fresh egg	63
Ground nutmeg	62
Ground lamb, cooked	61
Herring (without added oil)	59
Celery seed	58
Mustard seed	55
Coriander seed	54
Roasted chicken with skin	53
Salmon	52
Sardines	48
Cottage cheese	39

Note that many natural foods which have been downgraded nutritionally, such as eggs, meats, cheese, etc., contain no more fat than many processed foods. For example, some egg substitutes are higher in fat than fresh eggs. Natural foods are always better, whether they are high in fat, sugar or starch. Most people are familiar with natural, healthy foods rich in sugar and/or starch. These include corn, peas, beans, whole grains, fruits, and fruit juices. Now you can become familiar with how tasty, how appetizing, and how nutritious a high-natural fat diet really is — bon appetit!

CHAPTER 13
Two Weeks of Eating Right

E ating right means eating foods you tolerate well. Each individual will vary in what he/she tolerates best. This sample menu does not take into account any specific food allergies you may have. In order for the diet to be most effective, your food allergies must be determined. Even so, this diet does serve as an example of how eating a diet free of junk foods makes a major difference in how you feel. The elimination of junk foods from the diet is a major improvement in lifestyle. These harmful foods are so readily available, so habit-forming, and so convenient that anyone who consistently avoids them must be commended. This dietary program will give you the tools to accomplish this.

You will notice that these menus also eliminate foods naturally rich in carbohydrates, such as apples, rice, and whole-wheat bread. Even though these foods are wholesome and natural, it is better to go without them for the first 90 days. This will give your pancreas, liver, intestines, and adrenal glands a chance to rest from all the years of sugar overload.

Believe me, a diet low in sugars and starches can make all the difference in the world in how you feel. It is likely that you will notice a gradual increase in your energy or stamina and that you will not be as tired in the morning or evening. Another benefit is that you will be less sleepy during the day. There may also be a noticeable improvement in memory and concentration. With these and more benefits forthcoming, it is well worth it to practice these principles religiously for 90 days. After this time, you can introduce high-carbohydrate foods such as whole grains, potatoes, peas, corn, grapes, pears, apples, oranges, and honey.

However, introduce these foods gradually with your guide being whether or not adding them brings back any of your symptoms, such as fatigue, mental dullness, weight gain, indigestion, bloating, etc.

By the way, there is an interesting side effect from following this diet. You will probably lose weight. The longer you stick to it, the more weight you will lose. If you are already thin, or if you lose more weight than you need to, do not be concerned. Just add some carbohydrate-rich foods to the diet, such as potatoes, whole grains, fruits, or honey.

A word of caution: do not take the snacks lightly. They are probably the most important portion of the menu. These snacks prevent your blood sugar level from dropping. When blood sugar levels fall, cravings for sugary or starchy foods intensify to an uncontrollable degree. If you want this program to work, be sure to eat your snacks.

An asterisk (*) indicates that recipes can be found in the recipe section (Part II, Section 1).

ONE WEEK MENU
Day One

BREAKFAST

Scrambled Eggs Mediterranean Style*
one half cantaloupe or honeydew melon
glass of V-8 or tomato juice
vitamin supplements (take your vitamins three times a day with meals for best results — it is assumed you will continue taking them with each meal).

MID-MORNING SNACK: protein or Energy Shake*†

LUNCH

steamed vegetables with dip*
salad sprinkled with tuna or salmon — add as much as you like.
(olive oil and vinegar dressing)
one-half grapefruit
glass of unsweetened papaya or pomegranate juice

MID-AFTERNOON SNACK: almonds or pecans
Drink: Strawberry-Guava Punch*

† Diabetics, dieters, and those intolerant to carbohydrates should omit honey in the Energy Shake recipe.

DINNER

Roast Leg of Lamb*
squash, baked
green beans, steamed or cooked in a small amount of water
herbal tea
Dessert: Melon Smoothie*

Day Two

BREAKFAST

patty of ground turkey or chicken, cooked
two raw carrots
raw sunflower seeds, handful
grapefruit juice (fresh-squeezed is preferable)

MID-MORNING SNACK: protein powder in water or juice and/or hard-boiled egg

LUNCH

Italian Mushroom-Vegetable Soup*
salad with olive oil and vinegar
bowl of cottage cheese (or, cup of either kefir or home-made yogurt —
add diced melon or strawberries for extra taste.)
herbal tea

MID-AFTERNOON SNACK: Greek olives plus sliced vegetables
                         tomato juice or mineral water

DINNER

grilled salmon with herbs and lemon-butter (or olive oil)
Cole Slaw Salad (without added sugar)*
broccoli and/or cauliflower, steamed
kiwi fruit

Day Three

BREAKFAST

feta cheese omelet with 2 or 3 eggs (with or without spinach), basted in olive oil. †
one whole grapefruit, peeled
bowl of Greek olives
glass of V-8 or tomato juice

MID-MORNING SNACK: handful of pumpkin seeds, plus sliced vegetables
Drink: glass of mineral or purified water

LUNCH

one half baked chicken (preferably organic) plus spices
Carrots Piquant*
salad topped with zucchini and sliced onions, vinaigrette dressing
mineral or purified water

MID-AFTERNOON SNACK: slices of red and green peppers, handful of almonds (raw, or preferably, roasted with salt)
purified or mineral water

DINNER

lamb chops (second choice: veal chops)
salad topped with onions, Greek olives and feta cheese (olive oil, garlic and balsamic vinegar dressing)
spinach, steamed or boiled in small amount of water — drink juice.
small sweet potato (a special treat unless you are a diabetic, dieter, or are intolerant to carbohydrates)
glass of grapefruit juice

† Feta or goat's cheese is recommended because goat's milk products are much easier to digest than those made from cow's milk. In addition, while many people have developed allergies to cow's milk cheese, few are allergic to goat's milk cheese.

Day Four

BREAKFAST

Diced Zucchini in Olive Oil*
bowl of Greek olives
wedge of watermelon
glass of tomato or apricot juice

MID-MORNING SNACK: slices of feta or goat's cheese topped
with peanut butter
Drink: Carrot and Cream Cooler*

LUNCH

home-made Beef Stew (without potatoes)*
salad, topped with slices of cheese (olive oil, vinegar, and herb dressing)
herbal tea or decaffeinated coffee

MID-AFTERNOON SNACK: macadamia nuts or pumpkin seeds
herbal tea or tomato juice

DINNER

Grape Leaf Rolls without Rice (a very special treat)*
Mediterranean Salad*
Hummus*
sliced raw vegetables (carrots, romaine lettuce, carrots, and celery — dip
into the hummus)
purified water

Day Five

BREAKFAST

beefsteak, any type
one-half cantaloupe
cucumber slices, peeled
purified water

MID-MORNING SNACK: Protein Drink*
sliced vegetables (carrots, celery,
zucchini, turnips, etc.)

LUNCH

tuna salad in avocado boat
fruit garnish (melon, strawberries, grapefruit)
glass of fresh-squeezed or frozen vegetable juice (frozen juices are available at most health food stores)

MID-AFTERNOON SNACK: cup strawberry-flavored kefir or homemade yogurt**

DINNER

Green Bean Stew*
Brussels Sprout Carrot Celery Salad*
Diced Fruit in a Bowl (kiwi, papaya, strawberries, and melon)*
herbal tea or decaffeinated coffee (with real whipping cream if desired)

Day Six

BREAKFAST
sliced turkey breast
Grapefruit Medley*
glass carrot or grapefruit juice

MID-MORNING SNACK: Gazpacho Drink*
handful of almonds or pecans

LUNCH

fresh broiled fish or can of sardines
Lemon Cole Slaw*
steamed green vegetables (broccoli, green beans, Brussels sprouts, etc.)
kiwi fruit

MID-AFTERNOON SNACK: boiled egg or cup of yogurt
Strawberry-Almond Cooler*

** While I do not recommend milk, I do feel that fermented products made from *whole milk* are beneficial. Kefir is fermented milk which stays in a liquid state, while yogurt is more solid. A high quality kefir is now available in many supermarkets under the brand-name *Lifeway*. Most yogurts found in the supermarket are poor in quality. A recipe appears in the recipe section on how to make your own.

DINNER

stir fry chicken (or shrimp) sauteed in olive oil
(served on a bed of slivered almonds and pine nuts, lightly toasted)
carrot juice, fresh, canned or frozen
Diced Fruit in Bowl*

Day Seven

BREAKFAST

Diced Zucchini in Olive Oil plus two scrambled eggs*
one half cantaloupe or wedge watermelon
slices of tomatoes, cucumbers, and bell peppers. Salt if desired.
herbal tea

MID-MORNING SNACK: red pepper slices
                              handful of pistachios
                              mineral water

LUNCH

Pumpkin Soup*
Sauteed Brook Trout with Onions, Walnuts and Spices*
fresh vegetables, steamed (broccoli, cauliflower, cabbage, string beans,
etc.)

MID-AFTERNOON SNACK: slices of feta or Swiss cheese plus
                          Greek olives

DINNER

Kufta (Mediterranean Meatballs) with Sauce*
Mediterranean Yogurt and Cucumber Salad
Stuffed Cabbage Rolls (optional)*
tomato juice with lemon or lime

WEEK TWO
Day One

BREAKFAST

cheese slices topped with peanut, pecan, or almond butter (use goat's
cheddar or soy cheese found in health food stores)
celery and carrot sticks
herbal tea

MID-MORNING SNACK: roast beef slices
Drink: Cranberry Juice Creamy Surprise*

LUNCH

Poached Sweetbreads*
tossed salad (topped with Creamy Garlic-Avocado Dressing)*
purified water with twist of lemon or lime

MID-AFTERNOON SNACK: Protein Drink*
sliced vegetables

DINNER

Squash Soup*
White Fish in Lemon-Dill Sauce*
tomato slices topped with fresh or dried mint
Green Beans in Olive Oil (optional)*
carrot juice, canned, frozen, or fresh

Day Two

BREAKFAST

2 or 3 poached eggs
Herbed Turkey Sausage*
grapefruit juice, preferably fresh-squeezed

MID-MORNING SNACK: sliced chicken breast
Drink: Strawberry-Almond Cooler*

LUNCH

Salmon with Spring Vegetables and Hot Mustard*
Dilled Broccoli/Cauliflower Combo*
purified or mineral water with wedge of lime

MID-AFTERNOON SNACK: Nut and Olive Salad*
Chlorella Cooler (optional)*

DINNER

Artichoke Salad*
Simple Baked Onions*
Stuffed Lamb Loin*
Hummus*
Low-Carb Fruit Platter*

Day Three

BREAKFAST

Green Beans or Zucchini in Olive Oil* (add 1/4 pound ground lamb or
beef, if desired)
wedge watermelon
V-8 or tomato juice

MID-MORNING SNACK: chicken drumstick or breast
Drink: pink grapefruit juice

LUNCH

chef's salad topped with tuna, mackerel, or salmon
Pumpkin Soup*

MID-AFTERNOON SNACK: nut mix (pecans, almonds, pumpkin
and sunflower seeds)
glass purified or mineral water

DINNER

Onion Steak*
Italian-Mushroom Vegetable Soup*
Grilled Squash Medley*
slices of papaya and melon

Day Four

BREAKFAST

ground beef patty
Zucchini in Olive Oil*
glass of grapefruit juice

MID-MORNING SNACK: handful of olives
Protein Drink*

LUNCH

Spaghetti Squash Lasagna*
Sauteed Collard or Beet Greens*
purified water

MID-AFTERNOON SNACK: slices of lamb or beef roast
celery and carrot sticks
purified water

DINNER

Caper-Almond Salad*
Roast Duck with Melon Sauce*
Red Cabbage Curry*
Sesame-Garlic Tomatoes*
dessert: Watermelon Smoothie*

Day Five

BREAKFAST

Yogurt-Cucumber Salad*
nut butter on carrot and celery sticks
mineral or purified water

MID-MORNING SNACK: Blender Gazpacho*, Pro-Lecin
Nibblers™ (see appendix B).

LUNCH

Asparagus Soup*
Watercress Salad*
Crab Cakes*

MID-AFTERNOON SNACK: pecans or almonds
Melon Smoothie*

DINNER

Cabbage Soup*
Radish Salad*
Indian Chicken with Coriander Sauce*
mineral or purified water

Day Six

BREAKFAST

bowl cottage cheese with diced melon
Protein Drink*
V-8 or Very Veggie juice

MID-MORNING SNACK: handful pumpkin or squash seeds
grapefruit juice

LUNCH

tossed salad with olive oil and vinegar
Indian Coconut Curry*
bowl of strawberries or kiwi fruit
Cranberry Juice Creamy Surprise*

MID-AFTERNOON SNACK: slices of roast beef or lamb
carrot and celery sticks
purified or mineral water

DINNER

grilled salmon or tuna, with lemon-butter or olive oil
Lemon Cole Slaw*
Squash Stir-Fry*
Fruit 'n Nut Salad*
herbal tea

Day Seven

BREAKFAST
Scrambled Eggs Mediterranean Style*
1 whole grapefruit, peeled
glass tomato or V-8 juice

MID-MORNING SNACK: Nut and Olive Salad*
                           Protein Drink*

LUNCH
Lamb-Stuffed Artichokes*
Cabbage Soup*
Bermuda Onion/Beefsteak Tomato Delite*

MID-AFTERNOON SNACK: cucumber and tomato slices
                         slices of chicken or turkey breast
                         glass of grapefruit juice

DINNER
Turkey/Pumpkin Stew*
Sauteed Collard Greens*
sliced kiwi and strawberries
purified water

OH WHAT A WONDERFUL NUTRITIOUS MENU

This completes your first two weeks on a tasty, healthy menu. The menus serve to outline the basic principles of the diet. Use these principles, the recipes in Section II, and your own recipes to create additional weekly menus. Notice that you can eat fairly large quantities of food. In fact, if any of the menus are not filling enough, you can add additional salads or vegetable dishes as listed in the recipe section. Even if you are dieting, you need not starve. This is true as long as you eat *wholesome* foods, and as long as you don't cheat by adding *junk* foods. If you cut out the junk, you can enjoy the benefit of *eating until you are full* without risking your health or gaining excess weight.

NOW KEEP IT GOING

As always, a word of caution: many people, after a few weeks on the diet, hit a plateau where they feel so good and are so happy with their accomplishments that they decide to "reward" themselves. The reward, of course, is eating junk foods or possibly loading up on their allergic foods. The level of health within the body will determine how often one can "cheat" without sliding backwards. However, for most people, cheating on the diet will soon lead to a loss of whatever progress is made. The body is forgiving and can withstand a certain amount of abuse. However, most of you are reading this book because you have either noticed a decline in your health, or because you want to prevent any decline. Thus, I advise that you "hang in there" and keep the cheating to an absolute minimum.

IS IT GOOD TO EAT MEAT EVERY DAY?

I do not believe that in order to be healthy, you must eat meat every day. On the contrary, I think it is a good idea to occasionally go without meat. The reason foods such as beef, lamb, chicken, and fish are included so often is because they are *wholesome, unprocessed foods*. They are far more valuable food sources than the foods which commonly displace them such as doughnuts, muffins, breads, pasta, cookies, candies and soft drinks. In addition, in contrast to the foods just mentioned, fresh meats do not cause damage to the body. To be sure, there are some drawbacks to meats due to the addition of chemicals such as estrogens and antibiotics. A good compromise would be to buy "organic" meats. These are meats grown by farmers who do not use hormones or chemicals. It is interesting to note that Europeans will only allow the export of U.S.A. beef which is organic. We should demand the same.

However, I also am a firm believer in the health benefits of fasting. I suggest that at least twice each year you go several days without eating meat. Replace meats with extra quantities of fruits and vegetables. This will help "clean out" the digestive tract and give it the much needed rest it deserves.

CHAPTER 14
Conclusion

E ating right means using your common sense. It means following the laws of nature. I have illustrated how it is possible to eat wholesome foods of all types — meats, poultry, fish, fats, vegetables, grains, and fruits — without worry. Eating right is just as easy as eating wrong. Once you become accustomed to eating right, you will find it difficult to revert back to your old eating habits. This usually happens about 90 days after strictly following the dietary guidelines outlined in this book.

"Eating wrong" means putting things into your mouth that can harm your body. This includes all sorts of heavily processed foods. It includes white flour products, sugary desserts, sugar-ladened drinks, processed meats, as well as alcohol and cigarettes. While these foods and substances may taste good, provide a temporary feeling of elation, and/or have visual appeal, they are entirely devoid of nutritional value. In fact, with time, you will soon find that they become tasteless, and you may even come to abhor them.

Dying young could be a concern of the past, providing you follow the simple principles outlined in this book. Of course, no one is immune from natural disasters or accidental injury. I have only addressed the issue of premature deaths which are preventable — deaths from cancer, heart attacks, strokes, diabetes, neurological diseases, or any other potentially fatal degenerative disease. Such illnesses can kill rapidly. However, they may cause another form of "death" — a slow, writhing, painful existence which ends up eventually crippling or killing the individual.

161

Why get cancer, when you can prevent it? Why have a heart attack, when you can avoid it? Why develop arthritis, when you can abort it? What is the purpose of developing a paralyzing neurological disease, when it could be prevented? It just does not make sense to allow yourself to get these or other diseases when there is so much information available on health improvement and prevention.

The statistics are scary. The rate at which new diseases are developing is unprecedented in both modern and ancient history. Alzheimer's disease is a relatively recent phenomenon, as is AIDS. Heart disease is only a century old. Many cancers commonly seen today were never even heard of 40 years ago.

Bizarre neurological disorders such as multiple sclerosis, ALS (Lou Gerig's Disease), and muscular dystrophy are all 20th-century phenomenon. Diseases of the colon are modern day creations due largely to a diet low in fiber. Asthma and emphysema were relatively rare until the turn of the century. Obviously something has to change. Otherwise, it can only get worse.

What can be done to avoid being one of the statistics? The primary thing is to make some changes in the way you live. No doubt, the world is quickly becomming a toxic nightmare. There is only so much each individual can do about that. However, you can go into action to clean up *your* environment. There has to be some change in lifestyle. Something has to break.

I realize that change is not always easy. However, following some simple rules makes change a whole lot easier. Here are some rules of thumb for changing your immediate environment:

1. Make a law against eating anything that hurts you. Your body has a right to remain healthy. You have a responsibility to, above all, avoid harming it. This, by the way, is the Hippocratic Oath that all physicians must swear to abide by.

2. Prohibit yourself from using margarine, hydrogenated or partially hydrogenated fats. This would also include lard and shortening.

3. *Never* use commercial vegetable oils. Use instead extra-virgin olive oil or cold-pressed oils.

4. Cut your intake of sugar and sweets by at least three-fourths. Those with a major disease should eliminate sugar entirely. If you must have sweets, use honey. Be sure it is raw and unfiltered. Don't fool yourself into believing that sugars in the health food store are any better than white sugar.

5. Buy only wholesome foods for your home. Keep the junk out. Stock your refrigerator with fresh meats, milk products, eggs, vegetables and fruits.

6. Avoid buying food which is in a cardboard box. Some exceptions would include vegetables or fruits and whole grains. Most of these foods are highly processed and are adulterated with chemicals and additives.

7. Make every attempt to include foods grown without pesticides, herbicides, antibiotics, hormones, or other chemicals as part of your diet. These "organic" foods should make up at least 10% of your daily food intake. Another reason for needing the organic foods is that, pound for pound, they provide significantly more vitamins and minerals than commercial foods.

8. Supplement your diet with the minimal antioxidant program described in appendix D.

9. Clean up your water with a water purifier, a most important step.

10. Take a lot of antioxidants to counteract the air pollution, toxic chemicals, and radiation in the environment. The ozone crisis is another reason to take antioxidants.

I hope we can all work together to do something about the damage that is being done to the environment. I believe you must take care of yourself first. At least do that. Then, when we are all strong and healthy enough, we can go to battle for Mother Earth:

God made the earth beautiful; it is a bountiful resting place for man. He provided man with everything he needs; water to drink, food to eat, air to breath, herbs and medicines to heal.

Man, in his ignorance and possibly arrogance, has upset her fine chemistry, causing damage that is difficult, if not impossible to repair.

You know how immense the oceans are. As hard as it is to believe, these immense bodies of water are now polluted! The pollution of coastal waters is real. Those who have visited the east or west coast may have noticed there are few, if any, sea shells on the shores. As little as 30 years ago, these shells abounded on the beaches. Due to the pollution of the ocean and the shoreline by toxic wastes, radioactive chemicals, PCBs, agricultural run-off, sewage, and many other man-made insults, the number of gentle creatures which inhabited these shells and which have been found on the beaches for centuries have dwindled dramatically. Also, 1989 was the year of the dolphin — the year that over 6,000 of these precious creatures washed ashore, dead. The cause? A mysterious AIDS-like virus was to blame, so the newspapers reported. Believe me, the real cause was immune depression, leaving the dolphins wide open to infections by dangerous organisms — organisms which otherwise, could not have gained a foothold. This, for the dolphins, is the consequence of their "bathing" every second of the day in a sea of poison. This proves that despite the immense dilutional factor of all the water in the ocean, the toxic substances are effectively destroying portions of it. How can we go about cleaning up billions of gallons of salt water? It would be difficult, to say the least. The minimum that needs to be done is to stop any further dumping of chemical and human waste. We must hope that the earth herself will restore the oceans to normal.

You can see the enormity of it all. This is why I suggest that the focus be on the individual. In this book, you have been provided with several simple rules. The Time-Bombs have been discussed, and you are aware of the ones which can be avoided. Here are some other important keys to living right.

1. Never go a day without a bowel movement. If you haven't had one, the next step is to take a laxative, or mineral oil, right? Wrong. If necessary, resort to an enema. Add a teaspoon of liquid garlic extract to the enema, and retain it for as long as possible. This is better than taking harsh laxatives, and mineral oil removes essential fats and fat-soluble vitamins. Finding out what the problem is and fixing it is a better solution. Try some of the remedies listed in Part II of this book. Also, take sufficient amounts of fiber daily if you tend towards sluggish bowels. Herbal laxatives which are gentle in action, are often helpful. Ground flax seed is an excellent fiber supplement since it provides fiber and essential fatty acids, both of which improve colon function.

2. Do everything possible to move towards the bowel habits of a primitive: 2 to 4 large, soft, bulky movements per day.

3. Fast at least once per year. Go on a modified fast, abstaining from food and drink for at least 12 hours during the day. Do this for several days. Or try a juice fast, drinking only fresh-squeezed juices for 5-7 days. I do not recommend complete fasts using only water. I know this is done in some clinics and spas. Although a few may have benefited from these fasts, most of us would become too weak to withstand them.

4. Realize that life is a choice. You can choose to eat right, or you can continue to eat the way you do now. You can smoke cigarettes, drink alcohol to an excess, eat poorly, eat too much sugar, or you can choose to stop all of these health-robbing habits. This book has given you many of the tools necessary to replace the bad with the good.

5. Above all, be consistent. If you are going to fast, don't just do it once. Put a date on the calendar, and do it every year. Take your nutritional supplements on a daily basis, and follow the diet religiously. Take as many preventive measures as you can. By doing so, you may well save your life and avoid *dying young*.

PART II

Recipes
and
Remedies

PART II

Recipes for Eating Right

Entrees: Meats, Fish, Eggs and Poultry

BEEF STEW

1 cup water
1 lb. beef or veal, cut for stew (1/2 inch pieces)
1 celery stalk, diced
1/2 medium onion, chopped
2 carrots, sliced
1/2 cup fresh green beans, chopped in 1" sections
3 tablespoons rice bran (optional)
1 teaspoon salt
1 teaspoon pepper
1 bay leaf

Combine ingredients in Dutch oven or 2-quart casserole. Cover and bake in oven at 300 degrees for 2-1/2 hours. Remove bay leaf.
Makes 4 servings

TURKEY/PUMPKIN STEW

1 lb. turkey cooked
2 tablespoons olive oil or cold-pressed vegetable oil
1 green pepper, diced
1 red pepper, diced
1 cup pumpkin puree
4 cups chicken or turkey stock
1/2 onion, diced
3 1/2 cups fresh pumpkin, peeled and cubed
3 sage leaves, minced
parsley leaves, minced (for garnish)
pinch cayenne pepper
1 teaspoon honey (optional)

Cut turkey into cubes. In a Dutch oven, saute' turkey in oil until browned. Remove and place in a bowl. Saute' peppers and onions in same oil for 5 minutes. Mix pumpkin puree with stock, honey, and cayenne; then mix into pot with peppers and onions. Bring to a boil and add cubed pumpkin. Lower heat and add sage and turkey. Simmer for 30 to 45 minutes until all vegetables are tender. Serve garnished with parsley.
Makes 8 to 10 servings

CRACKERLESS MEATLOAF

1 lb. ground beef
3 tablespoons rice bran
1/4 cup onion, finely chopped
1/4 cup celery, finely chopped
1/4 cup sweet red pepper, finely chopped (optional)
1/2 teaspoon salt
1/8 teaspoon sage
1 6-oz. can tomato paste

Combine ingredients and mix well. Spoon into a 9 x 5 inch loaf pan. Press lightly. Bake at 325 degrees for one hour.
Makes 4 servings

SWEET AND TENDER LAMB STIR FRY

Have you ever heard of combining meat with fruit? This recipe does so in a unique way. Papaya contains special enzymes which aid in the digestion of meat. Garlic and onions help by improving the digestion of fat, in addition to preventing fat build-up in the blood. This extra-light, digestible meat dish represents an innovative method of preparing meat. Try it, you'll like it!

5 cloves garlic, finely chopped
1/2 large red onion, thinly sliced
1/2 lb. lamb meat, cut into 1" chunks
2 tablespoons extra virgin olive oil
1 teaspoon coriander seed, ground
1 cup papaya, chopped

In a medium non-stick skillet, combine garlic, onion, lamb, and oil. Lightly stir over medium high heat until lamb is browned. Add coriander and papaya and continue cooking just until papaya is hot.
Makes 2 to 4 servings

SALMON CAKES

8 ounces fresh or canned salmon (if canned, drain juice)
1/4 cup green pepper, chopped
1/4 cup oat or rice bran
1/4 cup vanilla yogurt (unsweetened), or plain yogurt
1/4 cup onion, chopped
1/4 teaspoon dried mustard
1/4 cup chopped celery
1 egg, beaten
salt to taste
dash of pepper

Combine all ingredients and spoon into four greased custard cups. Bake at 325 degrees for 30 minutes. Serve with sauce.

Sauce:
1/2 cup vanilla or plain yogurt (unsweetened)
1/2 cup cucumber, finely chopped (remove seeds and peel)
2 tablespoons chopped onion
1/2 cup sour cream
1/2 teaspoon dried dillweed or 1 teaspoon fresh dillweed

Combine ingredients in saucepan. Heat and pour over salmon cakes. *Makes 4 servings.*

KUFTA (Mediterranean meatballs)

5 lbs. ground round or hamburger (80% lean) or, 2-1/2 lbs. ground round with 2-1/2 lbs ground lamb.
1 tablespoon salt
1 teaspoon black pepper
1 tablespoon dried parsley or 2 tablespoons if fresh-chopped
1 tablespoon dried mint leaves or 2 tablespoons if fresh-chopped
3/4 cup finely chopped or shredded onions
2 eggs

In a large bowl, add meat, salt, black pepper, parsley, mint, and eggs. Mix all ingredients thoroughly with hands until the ingredients hold together. Make into balls with melon scooper or hand press to about one half the size of a walnut. Place in long cake pan (15 x 10) greased with a few drops of olive oil. Put the meatballs close together. Broil until brown, 3 to 4 minutes on each side. Cool and set aside.

Sauce:
2 fresh tomatoes, peeled and cubed (or 1 small can whole tomatoes, drained)
1 cup tomato sauce
1 large can V-8 or tomato juice
1 lb. ground round or 80% lean hamburger
2 medium onions, coarsely chopped
1 tablespoon salt
1 teaspoon black pepper
1/2 teaspoon garlic powder or 4 cloves fresh garlic, finely grated
1/4 cup olive oil
4 cups water

In a Dutch oven, saute' onions in olive oil for 2 to 3 minutes. Add hamburger and brown until the meat is no longer pink. Sprinkle meat mixture with salt, black pepper, and garlic. Cook on medium heat for about 7 minutes. Add fresh or canned tomatoes, tomato sauce, V-8, or tomato juice, and water. Bring to a boil. Turn to medium heat and cook for one half hour, stirring every 5 to 10 minutes. Add meatballs and cook an additional 5 minutes. Serve over toasted slivered almonds and pine nuts, or over brown rice. Rice can be used after your first 90 days on the diet.
Makes 20 servings

GRAPE LEAF ROLLS

3 lbs. coarse ground beef (80% lean)
2 tablespoons salt
1 teaspoon black pepper
1 teaspoon garlic powder
1 cup fresh chopped parsley (or 1/2 cup dried parsley flakes)
1/4 cup fresh chopped mint (or 1 tablespoon dried mint)
2 tablespoons olive oil
1 teaspoon garam masala (a spice sold in specialty stores —
    use All-Spice if this is not available)
1/2 cup green onions, chopped
1 teaspoon dried basil (or 1 tablespoon fresh chopped basil)
1/2 cup pinenuts (browned in a few drops of olive oil)
1 lb. jar grape leaves (sold in specialty stores and some supermarkets).

FILLING: Add together uncooked meat, salt, pepper, garlic, parsley, mint, olive oil, garam masala, green onions, basil, and pine nuts; mix all ingredients together until well blended.

HOW TO ROLL LEAVES: Drain grape leaves in a strainer. Take each leaf, stem facing you and lay it on a board. Spread 1 tablespoon of filling and roll tightly like a cigar with your fingers. Makes about 90 grape leaves. Takes approximately 1 hour to roll.

COOKING: If using a pressure cooker, cook all 90 rolls at once; otherwise, use two medium-sized pans.* Put small pieces of beef rib or chuck roast bones on the bottom. Place first layer of rolled grape leaves in a row. Criss-cross the remainder of the rows as you fill the pan. Once the pan is full, peel 6 whole cloves of garlic and put on top of the rolls. Sprinkle 1/4 teaspoon of salt and pour on 1 cup of lemon juice and 1/2 cup water. Cut one whole lemon in half, squeeze the juice, and put the lemon halves on top.

*If you are not using a pressure cooker, the recipe differs as follows: add 1-1/4 cup lemon juice and 3/4 cup water. Place heavy plate on top of rolls to help prevent them from breaking. Cover with lid and bring to full boil. Reduce heat to medium and cook for 25 minutes longer.

TO COOK IN PRESSURE COOKER: Put the tightly sealed lid on the pressure cooker and make sure the vent is open before putting the pressure knob on the lid. Turn on high heat. Let boil for 5 to 10 minutes after the pressure knob starts to squeak. Reduce heat to medium and cook for 15 minutes. Turn off stove. Let pressure cooker cool.

CAUTION IN SERVING: Do not open lid of pressure cooker when cooking or while it is still emitting steam. You can speed up the cooling process by running cold water over the cooker until steam disappears. Then it is safe to remove the lid. Serve warm as is or dip in hummus or home-made yogurt. Extras may be frozen.

SPAGHETTI SQUASH LASAGNA

All lasagna lovers will relish this wheat and noodle-free recipe. Spaghetti squash is different from other types of squash. When cooked, the flesh can be fluffed into strands which are very similar to noodles.

With this recipe, you receive the benefit of having noodles but without all the starch. Plus, spaghetti squash, pound for pound, is much higher in valuable nutrients such as beta carotene, potassium, calcium, magnesium, and vitamin C.

1 large spaghetti squash
1/2 lb. ground beef (85% lean)
1/2 teaspoon dried whole basil
1 clove garlic, crushed (or 1/8 teaspoon garlic powder)
1 eight oz. can whole tomatoes, drained
1 six oz. can tomato paste
1 ten oz. carton regular (not low fat) cottage cheese
1/4 teaspoon pepper
1/2 teaspoon salt
1/2 lb. sliced mozzarella cheese
1/4 cup fresh Parmesan cheese, grated
1 egg, beaten

Preheat oven to 350 degrees. Wash squash; pierce several times with fork and put on cookie sheet. Place in oven and bake for 1 hour or until soft. Once cool, cut squash in half and remove seeds. Using a fork, lift out the spaghetti-like strands. Measure out 4 cups of strands.

In a large, heavy skillet, cook ground beef until browned. Be sure to crumble well. Drain off grease. Add spices, tomato paste, tomatoes and simmer without covering for 30 minutes or more.

Mix together cottage cheese, Parmesan cheese, and egg in a bowl. Just as you would with regular lasagna, layer the three ingredients — the spaghetti squash, the cottage cheese mixture, and the ground beef mixture. Use a 12 x 8 x 2-inch baking or casserole dish. In a preheated oven, bake at 375 degrees for 25 to 30 minutes. Let stand for a few minutes and serve.

Makes 4 servings

LAMB-STUFFED ARTICHOKES

8 large globe artichokes
juice of 1 lemon
1 medium-sized onion, finely chopped
1 lb. ground lamb
1/4 cup pine nuts
1 tablespoon olive oil
2 teaspoons salt
1 tablespoon parsley, finely chopped
2 cups water
3 tablespoons butter
pepper

Wash artichokes thoroughly. Remove tough outer leaves and trim carefully around base just enough to look neat. Open leaves carefully with fingers to expose choke and remove this with a teaspoon. Drop prepared artichokes into a bowl of cold water with half the lemon juice added.

Saute' onion in olive oil until clear, then add pine nuts and stir over medium-low heat until lightly browned. Combine meat with onion and pine nut mixture, adding 1 teaspoon of salt and parsley. Add pepper to taste. Continue cooking until lamb is no longer pink.

Drain artichokes and fill centers with meat mixture, forcing in as much as they will take, and mounding meat at top. Arrange artichokes in a large pan, add water, and sprinkle remaining lemon juice over them. Sprinkle with an additional teaspoon of salt.

Cover and bring to a simmer. Gently simmer for 50 to 60 minutes until artichokes are tender. Drain off liquid into measuring cup. Keep artichokes hot.

SAUCE:

Melt butter. Add to one cup of drained water mixture. Pour over artichokes and serve.

Makes 8 servings

BEEF OR LAMB LIVER

1 lb. beef or lamb liver
1 large onion, sliced in rings
8 fresh mushrooms, sliced (or 1 medium can)
1/2 cup olive oil
salt
pepper
garlic powder

Slice liver, then cut slices in halves. Sprinkle onion and mushroom slices with salt, pepper and garlic powder.

In a large frying pan, add 1/4 cup olive oil, and heat on medium-high heat. Add liver and brown both sides. CAUTION: avoid overcooking the liver as most of its nutritional value will be lost. Remove liver and place on serving plate. Wipe oil out of pan and add the other 1/4 cup oil. Brown onions and mushrooms. Place mushrooms and onions on top of liver and serve immediately.

Makes 4 servings

GREEN BEAN AND LAMB STEW

2 lbs. lamb roast (although lamb is preferable, you may use chuck roast) trim visible fat and cut into cubes
4 cloves fresh garlic, diced
1 large onion diced
8 fresh tomatoes (or 1 large can of whole tomatoes), chopped
3 lbs. fresh or frozen green beans
1 small can tomato sauce, unsweetened
2 teaspoons salt
1 teaspoon pepper
1/4 cup olive oil.

Wash and cut beans into pieces, being sure to remove stems. Put olive oil into 6-quart pot and heat for one minute. On medium heat, add meat cubes, salt, pepper and brown for ten minutes or until there is no visible redness. Add onions and garlic and stir constantly for 2 minutes. Add tomatoes, and if canned, reserve juice. Continue stirring for 1 to 2 minutes. Add tomato sauce and reserved tomato juice. Stir and add green beans. **Note:** If you are using frozen beans, cook sauce on medium heat 1/2 hour before adding beans. Water may be added, if needed. Garnish with parsley.

Makes 8 servings

WHITE FISH IN LEMON-DILL SAUCE

White fish of any type (whitefish, flounder, walleye, orange roughy, etc.) will fit well into this recipe. White fish itself is an excellent choice, since it is rich in certain fish oils known as omega-3 fatty acids. These help improve circulation and prevent degenerative disease.

2 tablespoons butter
1 tablespoon fresh lemon juice
5 slices lemon with rind
1 tablespoon freshly chopped dill (or 3/4 tablespoon dried dill)
1 small onion, sliced thin
1 lb. fresh or frozen white fish fillets

Heat butter, dill, lemon juice, salt, and onion in large skillet over medium-low heat; saute' for about three minutes. Add white fish and lemon slices; cover and cook for 7 to 9 minutes and baste occasionally. Pour sauce over fish and serve.
Makes 2 to 4 servings

SALMON WITH SPRING VEGETABLES AND HOT MUSTARD

Are you happy to hear that mustard is good for you, and that it belongs to a family of vegetables known to prevent cancer? Brown mustard is a nutritious addition to food selections. It is high in certain vitamins as well as essential fatty acids and protein. Coarse brown mustard is the preferred type, since it undergoes the least amount of processing.

1 lb. Alaskan salmon
2-3 tablespoons butter
1 cup julienned carrots
1 cup finely julienned white part of leek
1 cup julienned (peeled) celery
1/2 teaspoon black pepper
1/2 cup julienned zucchini
1 cup fish stock
salt
1/3 cup all-natural brown mustard

In a large saucepan or skillet, melt butter. Scatter half the carrots, leeks, celery, and zucchini in pan and turn to medium heat. Sprinkle pinch of salt. Place salmon fillets into the pan beside the vegetables, and add pepper and the remaining vegetables. Slowly pour in fish stock. Cover and simmer for 5 to 6 minutes only. Remove from heat. In a small saucepan, add 1 tablespoon butter and melt. Add mustard and cook until hot. Serve over fish, or as a dip for fish and/or vegetables.
Makes 4 servings

POACHED HADDOCK PORTUGUESE STYLE

1 lb. haddock fillets
1 medium onion, finely chopped
1/4 cup fresh parsley, finely chopped
2 tablespoons tarragon vinegar
2 cloves garlic, crushed
1/2 teaspoon thyme
3 tomatoes, diced
1 teaspoon olive oil

Place fish in water in a heavy pan or electric skillet and cover with the remaining ingredients. Bring mixture to a boil, then cover and simmer for 10 to 12 minutes. Remove the fish carefully so it doesn't break apart and keep warm by covering with foil while the sauce is heated and boiled down. Once reduced by half, pour sauce while it is hot over the fish and serve.
Makes 4 servings

SAUTEED BROOK TROUT WITH ONIONS, WALNUTS AND SPICES

4 whole brook trout, boned
2 limes (use 1/4 cup vinegar if you are citrus sensitive)
3 medium onions, peeled and cut into 8 wedges each
1 cup walnuts, coarsely chopped
1/4 cup olive oil
1/2 teaspoon ground turmeric
1/4 teaspoon ground cinnamon
1/4 teaspoon ground cumin
salt and pepper
1/4 cup cold-pressed vegetable oil (peanut, sunflower, or safflower)

Squeeze the juice of one lime and set aside. Thinly slice the other lime and set slices aside. In a medium-sized saucepan, heat olive oil over low heat. Add onions and saute' for 10 to 15 minutes until limp but do not brown. Remove the pan from heat and stir in walnuts, turmeric, cinnamon, cumin, and 1/2 teaspoon salt. Set aside and keep warm.

Wash trout under cold water and pat dry. Lightly sprinkle the cavity and skin with salt and pepper. In a large skillet, heat vegetable oil over medium-high heat but be careful not to burn the oil. Add trout, 2 at a time, cooking until golden brown and cooked through.

To serve, spoon onion mixture into the cavity of each trout, pour remaining sauce over the trout and garnish with lime juice and slices.
Makes 4 servings

STUFFED LAMB LOIN

3 tablespoons olive oil
¼ cup onion, finely chopped
2 garlic cloves, crushed
1 cup spinach, shredded
¼ cup fresh parsley, finely chopped
¼ cup fresh basil, shredded
2 tablespoons sundried tomatoes, finely chopped
2 tablespoons pine nuts (or sunflower seeds), chopped
2 teaspoons lemon pepper
1 teaspoon salt
½ cup crumbled feta cheese
1¾ to 2 lbs. fresh lamb sirloin roast, boned

In a medium skillet, heat 2 tablespoons olive oil; saute' onion and garlic for 2 to 3 minutes. Mix in spinach, parsley, basil, sundried tomatoes, pine nuts and 1 teaspoon of lemon pepper. Cook additional 2 to 3 minutes or until spinach and parsley are wilted. Mix in feta cheese; set aside. Preheat oven to 325 degrees. Remove all visible fat from meat. Make a slice one half way through the meat lengthwise down the center. Cover with plastic wrap and with meat mallet, pound to 1-inch thick. Place filling down center of meat; roll and tie with string at 2-inch intervals.

Brush with 1 tablespoon olive oil and sprinkle with 1 teaspoon lemon pepper and salt. Place on rack and roast to desired degree of doneness. This can be tested with a thermometer. For medium-rare, roast for 1½ hour (150 degrees), or for medium, roast for an additional 10 minutes (160 degrees).
Makes 6 to 8 servings

INDIAN CHICKEN WITH CORIANDER SAUCE

2 onions, peeled and quartered
10 tablespoons olive oil or cold-pressed peanut or sesame oil
3 whole skinless, boneless breasts of chicken (preferably organic)
1/4 cup slivered almonds
3 tablespoons ground coriander
1 teaspoon ground cardamom
1 piece fresh ginger, about 2 inches long, peeled
2 cups plain yogurt
2/3 cup fresh coriander leaves (or 2 tablespoons dried)
1 teaspoon black pepper, preferably freshly ground
1/4 teaspoon salt
1 cup water
sliced almonds (to garnish)

Using a food processor, finely chop the onions and set aside. Use it again to finely chop the coriander leaves and ginger; set aside. Heat 2 tablespoons oil in a large, deep skillet over medium heat. Add chicken breasts and cook until lightly brown (about one minute each side). Remove and set aside.

Add the remaining oil and heat; add onions and cook until limp, but not brown. Stir in 1/4 cup almonds and cook for 2 additional minutes. Next, add coriander - ginger mixture; mix well. While still on medium heat, add the rest of the spices, yogurt, reserved chicken breasts, and 1 cup of water; bring to a boil over high heat. Cover and reduce to a simmer for 25 to 30 minutes or until the chicken is thoroughly cooked. Remove from heat and let stand for 30 minutes to enhance flavor.

Reheat chicken mixture over low heat while, at the same time, sauteing the remaining almonds in a teaspoon of oil (use a small skillet) until lightly browned. Serve by pouring sauce over chicken and topping with almonds.
Makes 3 servings

BROILED CHICKEN PIECES WITH SPICES

1 whole chicken, cut into pieces (leave skin on)
2 tablespoons olive oil
2 cloves garlic, sliced (or 1/4 teaspoon garlic powder)
1/2 teaspoon salt
1/8 teaspoon pepper
paprika

Place chicken pieces on cookie sheet. Add olive oil, garlic, salt, and pepper to a small bowl and mix. Spread mixture over front and back of chicken pieces. Sprinkle paprika on back side. Lay chicken with the skin down and place into broiler. Broil on each side until brown (about 5 minutes); sprinkle paprika on front side after turning over. Place into preheated oven (350 degrees) and cook for an additional 25 to 30 minutes. Baste juices or additional oil over chicken if necessary.
Makes 4 servings

INDIAN COCONUT CURRY

Coconut milk is very filling due to its high fat content. Try this all-vegetable curry for a change in pace from meat-containing entrees.

2 cups fresh coconut, cut in 1/2 inch cubes (or, 1 cup canned coconut milk)
1 cup water
1 cup chopped onion
1/2 cup chopped green pepper
1/4 cup peanut oil (cold-pressed)
1 teaspoon curry powder
1/4 teaspoon salt
1/2 teaspoon cardamom seed, crushed
2 cups cauliflower
1 cup broccoli
1/4 cup fresh-squeezed lemon juice
2 cups sweet potatoes, cubed (optional)

Add to blender coconut and water, blending at high speed until smooth. Strain through two thicknesses of cheesecloth, squeezing out liquid. (You have just made fresh coconut milk). In a large, heavy skillet, heat oil and saute' onions and green pepper until clear. Add all spices. Next, add sweet potato, cauliflower, broccoli, and water as needed. When vegetables are tender, add coconut milk and lemon juice. Cover, let stand for 5 minutes and serve.
Additional suggestions: for extra vegetable protein, pour curry over toasted pine nuts or slivered almonds. A fitting drink would be any of the creamy coolers which are listed in the drink section.

The next four recipes are compliments of Chefs' Felice Martinelli, Steven Dunn, and Robert Jones of *Amourette*, located in Palatine, Illinois.

CRAB CAKES

8 oz. fresh crab meat, shredded
1 whole egg
1 teaspoon brown mustard
2 tablespoons of mayonnaise (sugar-free brands made with cold-pressed
   oils are available in health food stores)
dash of salt
dash of white pepper
dash of Tabasco sauce
1 teaspoon rice bran
1 teaspoon clarified butter

In a large bowl, combine crab meat, egg, and mustard; mix thoroughly. Add mayonnaise and mix until mixture is paste-like. Add salt and pepper, rice bran and Tabasco sauce.

To cook, mold crab mixture in the size of a silver dollar. Saute' in skillet with clarified butter until golden brown on both sides. Serve with a cayenne-flavored mayonnaise or mustard.

Makes 2 servings

ROAST DUCK WITH MELON SAUCE

1 3-1/2 to 4 lb. duckling
1/3 cup vegetable oil (cold-pressed)
1 teaspoon dried thyme
2 bay leaves
1/4 teaspoon salt
black pepper

Cut off excess fat from around duck body. Crush bay leaves and sprinkle inside duck cavity. Add thyme, salt, and sprinkle pepper inside cavity. In a large pan, heat the oil and sear the duck first on the bottom, then turn over and sear the side until light brown (this will prevent the duck from sticking to the pan while roasting). Drain excess oil.

Heat oven to 425 degrees, and place duck in oven for 1-1/2 hours.

MELON SAUCE

1 honeydew melon, remove seeds and retain juice
1 tablespoon shallots, chopped

2 tablespoons honey (optional)
2 tablespoons butter

Puree melon and set aside. Heat butter in saucepan and add shallots; saute' until limp. Add pureed melon and honey; simmer for 10 to 15 minutes. Strain in a fine sieve and try to get all the juice out by pressing down with a ladle. Return juice to pan; bring to a boil. Reduce heat and cook until mixture thickens.

Cut roasted duck from carcass. Spoon sauce over duck and garnish with melon balls.

Makes 4 to 6 servings

POACHED SWEETBREADS

1 lb. of sweetbreads (soaked in cold water overnight)
1-1/2 qt. water
1/2 onion
1 small carrot, chopped
1 rib celery, chopped
1 leek end (use white only)
bay leaf
2 sprigs of fresh thyme (optional)
juice of one lemon
cracked black pepper

Add all ingredients together in pot (except sweetbreads). Bring to boil. After boiling for a few minutes, add sweetbreads. When water comes back to a slow simmer, remove from heat and let cool. Leave ingredients in stock and refrigerate.

SAUCE:

1/2 to 3/4 cup balsamic vinegar
3-1/2 cups olive oil or cold-pressed vegetable oil (sesame, corn, or sunflower)
1/4 cup shallots, minced
1 egg yolk (use 1 tablespoon of pureed avocado if you have an egg yolk allergy)
2 tablespoons of brown (all-natural) mustard
1/4 cup fresh parsley, chopped
1 teaspoon salt
1/4 teaspoon white pepper
2 tablespoons water (if needed)

Add all ingredients in mixing bowl except oil and vinegar. Now add small amount of vinegar and mix well. Pour in oil, a little at a time while whisking the mixture rapidly to form an emulsion. When it starts to thicken, add a little more vinegar to thin. Now add the oil and water alternately until all is in bowl. If mixture is too thick or strong, add water to thin or lighten flavor.

TO SERVE: Heat sweetbreads in stock until hot and remove. Strain vegetables and place over sweetbreads. Pour on sauce as desired, and serve.
Makes 4 servings

ONION STEAK

1/4 cup freshly squeezed onion juice
1/2 large onion, sliced
1/4 teaspoon garlic powder (or 2 cloves garlic, crushed)
1/2 teaspoon salt
2 steaks of your choice

Marinate steaks in mixture of onion juice, salt, and garlic powder for at least 2 hours. When ready, cook in oven, or fry in skillet on medium heat. Caution: do not overcook the meat as this will reduce its digestibility and destroy most of its nutritional value. Fry onion slices in skillet on medium-low heat for 3 to 4 minutes, or until clear. Top steaks with onions and serve. Add sauteed mushrooms, if desired.
Makes 2 servings

GRILLED MARINATED STEAK WITH RED PEPPER SAUCE

3 tablespoons olive oil
1 medium red onion, diced
3 cloves garlic, chopped
1 small fresh hot chili pepper, seeded and finely chopped
4-6 large sweet red bell peppers
3 to 4 lbs. New York strip or sirloin steak
1/8 teaspoon salt
1/8 teaspoon black pepper

MARINADE:

1-1/2 cup olive oil
1/2 cup balsamic vinegar
3 sprigs fresh thyme

RED PEPPER SAUCE: Over an open flame, sear red bell peppers, turning with tongs to scorch skin on all sides (or broil, turning frequently). Place roasted peppers in paper bag, folding the top closed. Preheat oven to 200 degrees and cook peppers in oven for 50 minutes. Remove peppers and cool with running water. At the same time, remove any burned outer skin. Core the peppers, discarding core and seeds. Chop coarsely. In a food processor or blender, puree peppers until smooth.

In a non-stick skillet, heat olive oil and saute' onion, garlic, and chili pepper until chili pepper is softened (4 to 5 minutes). Set aside.

In a small bowl combine bell pepper puree with onion-garlic mixture. Season with salt and pepper. Let sauce stand 2 hours at room temperature to blend flavors.

In a large pan combine marinade ingredients. Add steaks and turn to coat. Let stand at room temperature for at least 2 hours (or for 8 to 12 hours in refrigerator). Cook steaks over grill until medium or medium rare. Serve topped with heated pepper sauce.
Makes 10 to 12 servings

ROAST LEG OF LAMB

1 leg of lamb (or lamb shoulder)
1/4 cup olive oil
4 cloves garlic, crushed
1/2 lemon
1/2 orange
1/4 teaspoon salt
1/4 teaspoon pepper
2 onions, peeled and quartered
2 stalks celery, cut into 3 inch pieces
1 cup water

Place leg of lamb in a roaster. Along side, add quartered onion and celery. In a bowl, add juice of lemon and orange along with crushed garlic, olive oil, salt and pepper. Mix for a few seconds. Pour mixture over meat, making sure to cover meat evenly. Add water to the bottom of roaster.

In a preheated oven (350 degrees), heat uncovered for about 2 hours. Check roast frequently during this period, basting it in its juices. At the 2 hour interval, baste roast with 2 tablespoons of olive oil. Cover and cook for an additional 3 hours (a total of 5 hours) and serve.
Makes 6 servings

MEATBALLS ON SQUASH ALMONDINE

1 large winter (spaghetti) squash
1/2 cup slivered almonds
1/2 cup onion, chopped
6 cloves of garlic, crushed
1 lb. hamburger meat (85% lean) or 1/2 lb. ground beef and 1/2 lb. ground lamb.
1/2 cup fresh parsley, finely chopped
1/4 cup green or red peppers, chopped
1/4 cup celery, chopped
1/4 cup capers (optional)
1/2 cup rice bran or 1/2 cup cooked wild rice
1/2 teaspoon salt (or preferably 1 teaspoon sea salt)
1 tablespoon olive oil
2 16 oz. cans tomato sauce (unsweetened)

Add onions, garlic, parsley, peppers, celery, capers, salt, bran (or wild rice) and hamburger together in large mixing bowl. Gently mix hamburger and ingredients with hands until all are well combined. Make into large meatballs. Brown meatballs in heavy skillet in olive oil. Drain oil and fat from meatballs and discard. Add tomato sauce, and simmer until meatballs are light pink in the center.

Bake squash until outside is soft. Scoop out interior and set aside. In a small skillet heat a small amount of olive oil and add slivered almonds. Cook until browned and combine with squash. Serve meatballs and sauce over spaghetti squash and almonds. You may also serve over wild rice if spaghetti squash is not available.
Makes 6 to 8 servings

SCRAMBLED EGGS MEDITERRANEAN STYLE

For the egg lover this is a wonderful treat. If at all possible, try to use farm-fresh eggs.

3 eggs, extra-large
1/4 cup olive oil
1/4 cup green onions, diced (use entire onion)
1 clove garlic, crushed

Crack eggs into bowl. Using a non-stick skillet, heat olive oil on medium-low heat, and add onions and garlic. Saute' until lightly browned. Add eggs and scramble. Avoid cooking eggs excessively, as this will reduce their nutritional value. Serve hot.
Makes 2 servings

SOUPS

ASPARAGUS SOUP

1 lb. asparagus stalks
3 cloves garlic, minced
4 green onions, diced
1 tablespoon olive oil
2 cups water or chicken stock
1 tablespoon fresh parsley, chopped
2 teaspoons lemon juice, fresh
1 teaspoon ground coriander
dash of white pepper
1/4 teaspoon salt

Slice off hard ends of asparagus stalks, and chop the rest into 1 inch chunks. Reserve the tips. In a saucepan, saute' onions and garlic in olive oil over medium-low heat until limp. Add water or stock, asparagus, parsley, lemon juice and spices. Cook until asparagus is tender. Put in electric blender and blend until smooth. Return to pan and add reserved asparagus tips; cook until hot and serve.
Makes 4 to 6 servings

PEANUT BUTTER-TOMATO SOUP

1/2 cup chopped onion
1 cup diced celery
2 cups stewed tomatoes
2 tablespoons butter (use olive or peanut oil if you are butter-sensitive)

2 tablespoons pure peanut butter
4 cups water
1 teaspoon salt, or to taste

Press tomatoes through a colander or process in blender. Saute' onion and celery in butter in a heavy skillet until tender. Thoroughly mix tomatoes with peanut butter and add along with other ingredients. Simmer until well-blended and serve.
Makes 6 to 8 servings

PUMPKIN SOUP

1 cup chopped green onions (include stems)
2 cups mashed, cooked pumpkin (or one 16-oz. can)
2 tablespoons chives
3 cups chicken stock
1 cup grated carrots
1/4 teaspoon nutmeg
1/2 teaspoon ginger
dash of pepper
1/3 cup whipping cream
1/2 cup water
2 tablespoons fresh parsley, chopped

Saute' onions in a non-stick pan until limp. Add remaining ingredients except whipping cream and parsley. Cover and simmer for 20 minutes. Stir in whipping cream and serve. Garnish each bowl with fresh parsley.
Makes 6 to 8 servings

ITALIAN MUSHROOM-VEGETABLE SOUP

1/2 tablespoon basil
2 tablespoons olive oil
1 large onion, chopped
2 large cloves garlic, minced
3 ribs celery, sliced
2 cups mushrooms, sliced
1 tomato, finely chopped

1 large carrot, finely chopped
1 can tomato sauce, unsweetened
1 can tomato juice from canned tomatoes
4 cups chicken stock
4 cups various sliced vegetables (such as zucchini, yellow squash, and
    green beans)

Saute' onion, garlic, celery, and carrot in olive oil until almost soft.
Add mushrooms and cook until barely tender. Add liquids, vegetables,
and basil. Bring to a boil and simmer until vegetables are tender.
Makes 12 servings

CABBAGE SOUP

3 cups cabbage, coarsely chopped
3 cups tomato juice
1 cup water
1 carrot, peeled and sliced
2 tablespoons fresh parsley, chopped
1/2 cup onion, chopped
1/4 cup red or green pepper, chopped
1/2 cup celery, chopped (include leaves)
1/8 teaspoon salt
dash of pepper
dash of basil or thyme to taste

Bring juice and water to boil. Add vegetables and seasonings. Boil
again and simmer for 15 to 20 minutes.
Makes 6 servings

SQUASH SOUP

3 pounds winter or butternut squash
3 tablespoons butter
1/3 cup chopped onion
1 clove garlic, crushed
1 teaspoon coriander, ground
1/4 teaspoon ground cardamom
1/2 teaspoon salt
chopped parsley
3 cups water or stock

Simmer squash in water or stock 10 minutes or until tender. Set aside. Saute' onion and garlic in butter until soft. Stir in seasonings and add to squash mixture. Add all ingredients (except parsley) into blender and process until smooth. Make into two batches if necessary. Place in saucepan and heat. Garnish with chopped parsley and serve.
Makes 4 servings

WATERCRESS-TOMATO SOUP

2 tablespoons butter or olive oil
1 leek, sliced
1/4 cup chopped onion
1 teaspoon minced garlic (fresh), or 1/2 teaspoon garlic powder
2 cups canned, peeled whole tomatoes (cut into pieces)
1-1/2 cups chicken stock
1 bunch watercress, stems removed
2 tablespoons fresh parsley (chopped)
dash pepper
salt to taste

In a medium sized saucepan, saute' leek, onion, and garlic in butter or olive oil. Cover and cook over low heat for 10 minutes. Add tomatoes and chicken stock and bring to a boil. Reduce heat and simmer for 15 to 20 minutes. Add watercress, parsley, and spices. Simmer for an additional 5 to 10 minutes and serve.
Makes 4 servings

NOODLE-LESS MINESTRONE

3 large onions, finely chopped
4 tablespoons olive oil
1 quart vegetable stock
1 quart water
1 large can tomatoes, chopped
3/4 teaspoon garlic salt
3/4 teaspoon celery salt
1/2 teaspoon basil
1/2 teaspoon oregano
1/4 teaspoon thyme
1 cup zucchini, sliced in julienne strips

Saute' onions and vegetables in oil. Add stock and water; bring to a boil. Add tomatoes and spices. Simmer for 10 minutes. Sprinkle with Parmesan cheese, if desired.
Makes 10 servings

HEALTHY HEART SOUP (A Cold Soup)

This soup is good for the heart because it is rich in three heart-nourishing nutrients — carnitine, coenzyme Q-10, and selenium. Avocados are the richest known plant source of carnitine, and garlic is an excellent natural source of coenzyme Q-10. Garlic is also high in the heart-saving mineral selenium, especially if it is grown on selenium-rich soil.

2 ripe avocados
2 large cloves garlic, crushed
1 tablespoon olive oil
1-1/2 tablespoons red wine vinegar
2 ripe tomatoes, peeled
3/4 cup Very Veggie (spicy type)* (V-8 juice may be substituted)
1/2 teaspoon sea salt
1/2 medium white onion cut in large pieces
2 tablespoons green onion tops, chopped

Peel avocados and cut into pieces. Add avocado to blender and blend until smooth. Coarsely chop tomatoes and onions and place in blender. Add garlic, salt, olive oil, Very Veggie juice, and vinegar and blend entire mixture until smooth. Serve as is or chilled. Garnish with green onion tops.
Makes 4 servings

CHICKEN "CURE A COLD" SOUP

This soup contains all sorts of ingredients useful in relieving the symptoms of colds—and some which can help the immune system cure it. The soup is high in vitamins A and C, plus it contains lots of garlic and onions—nature's antibiotics. Chicken broth and fat provide essential

---

*This recipe works best with Very Veggie, a spicy, natural vegetable juice made by R.W. Knudsen. Very Veggie may be found in the health food section of some supermarkets and in most health food stores. If you cannot find it, use V-8 juice and add 1 crushed, fresh chili pepper.

fatty acids which also have antibiotic-like action. The Cure a Cold Soup is far and above any over-the-counter medicine or remedy for providing relief. Watch your sinuses and breathing passages open up after eating this hearty, nourishing soup.

18 cloves garlic, crushed or finely diced
1 extra-large yellow onion, diced
2 teaspoons Hungarian paprika
2 teaspoons coriander
2 teaspoons salt
1 teaspoon lemon pepper
3 bay leaves
½ cup parsley, minced
4 medium-sized carrots, peeled and diced into large chunks
²/₃ cup celery, diced
1 large red sweet pepper, cored and diced
1 cup cooked Brussels sprouts, whole. Remove any discolored outer leaves
1 cup fresh or frozen green beans, stems removed
½ medium-sized turnip, peeled and diced
½ chicken, whole with skin on

Wash chicken thoroughly. In a large pot, place chicken in water and boil for 20 to 30 minutes. Skim top layer off water. Add garlic, lemon pepper, coriander, bay leaves, salt, and onion; continue cooking over reduced heat. Add vegetables and cook for an additional 10 to 20 minutes or until flavors blend.
Makes 4 to 6 servings

HOT OR COLD TOMATILLO SOUP

Tomatillos are also known as strawberry tomatoes. They are a tasty and more wild version of regular tomatoes. Tomatillos are native to Mexico and are commonly used in Mexican cooking. They are low in calories and high in fiber.

6 tomatillos, sliced.
¼ cup green pepper, diced
1 large red sweet pepper, chopped in large pieces
4 cloves garlic, finely sliced
1 cup Very Veggie
¼ cup green onions, diced (whites and greens)

dash cardamom (optional)
½ teaspoon salt
2 teaspoons olive oil

In a medium skillet, saute' over low heat garlic, onions, and all vegetables in olive oil until tender, being careful not to over-cook. Add Very Veggie, salt and cardamom and cook until hot. Serve immediately or refrigerate and serve cold.
Makes 2 servings

SALADS

RADISH SALAD

This salad is especially good for those with digestive problems. Radishes contain substances which stimulate digestive juices and help heal the lining of the stomach and intestines. In addition, they are useful for the cardiac patient or for anyone with a concern or family history of cancer, since they are a rich natural source of the mineral selenium. Try to get radishes grown in states with selenium-rich soil, such as the Dakotas, Iowa, Missouri, Kansas, Nebraska, Arizona, Colorado, Oklahoma, Texas, and some parts of California.

1/2 cup red radishes, diced
1/2 cup daikon radish, diced
red radish sprouts (optional), handful
1/2 cup cucumbers, chopped
1/2 cup red onion, chopped
1 cup cherry tomatoes, sliced in quarters
1/4 cup balsamic vinegar
3 tablespoons olive oil
2 tablespoons fresh parsley, finely chopped

Combine all ingredients into salad bowl and gently toss. Serve as is or topped with crumbled feta cheese.

WATERCRESS SALAD

Watercress has long been known to have valuable medicinal and nutritional values. As indicated by its name, watercress grows naturally in water. It has a very high water content (93%) and almost no calories. A one cup serving of watercress provides almost as much calcium as a cup of milk. In addition, it is low in phosphorus, which makes it a better calcium source. Watercress is also very rich in vitamins A and C. It should be on the top of your list of anti-cancer foods.

10 sprigs of watercress
1/2 head lettuce, shredded
1 tablespoon chopped sweet red pepper
1/2 cup diced cucumber
8 radishes, thinly sliced
1/2 cup grated goat's milk cheese or white cheddar cheese
onion or garlic salt to taste

Toss all ingredients together in a bowl just before serving. Use a dressing of your choice.
Makes 4 to 6 servings

NUT AND OLIVE SALAD

If you are nuts over nuts, you will love this salad. Nuts are an excellent addition to salads, because they are crunchy and are more filling than vegetables alone. Olives are also very filling due to their high fat content.
12 large black or green olives, pitted
2 tablespoons walnuts, chopped in large chunks
2 tablespoons pecans
1 tablespoon raw or roasted sunflower or pumpkin seeds
1 head lettuce, chopped or torn
1/4 cup chopped celery
1/4 cup finely shredded red cabbage
1/4 cup shredded carrots
parsley sprigs (as garnish)
salt to taste

Toss lettuce and vegetables in large bowl. Add salt to taste. Mix nuts in a separate bowl. Put salad mixture in salad bowls, and top with nuts. Chill or serve as is with or without a dressing of your choice.
Makes 6 to 8 servings

BERMUDA ONION/BEEFSTEAK TOMATO DELIGHT

This salad really hits the spot, particularly on a hot, summer day. Both onions and tomatoes are cooling, as is parsley. Try it as part of your dinner menu or as a snack by itself.

4 extra thick (1/3 inch) slices of Bermuda onion
2 large tomatoes, cut in extra thick slices
2 tablespoons fresh parsley, chopped (or 1 tablespoon parsley flakes)
1/3 cup goat's feta (crumbled), or shredded Swiss cheese
1 clove garlic, crushed
1/4 teaspoon black pepper
dash salt
olive oil and vinegar

On two plates, alternate a layer of tomatoes and onions at an angle. Mix parsley, garlic, salt, and pepper with olive oil and vinegar (balsamic and tarragon would be excellent choices), and pour over plates. Top with cheese and a few pine nuts, if desired.
Makes 2 servings

VARIETY LETTUCE SALAD WITH PINE NUTS AND GOAT'S CHEESE

When making a salad, it is always best to use several types of vegetables. By using several varieties of lettuce, the nutritional value of the salad increases. Pine nuts are one of the finest vegetable sources of high-quality protein, and they are easily digested.

1/2 cup pine nuts
1/2 lb. green beans
1 head radicchio lettuce
1 head of Boston lettuce
1/2 head Bibb lettuce
1/2 head romaine lettuce
1/2 lb. goat or feta cheese
1 quart water
1/2 teaspoon salt

Wash vegetables and lettuce thoroughly in cold water, drying off any water. Trim edges of green beans. Preheat oven to 400 degrees. Place pine nuts on cookie sheet and put in oven for 6 minutes to toast, shaking pan several times.
Bring water to a boil and add salt. Add the green beans and cook until the beans are tender but still crisp (about 4 to 6 minutes). Drain, refresh under cold water, and set aside.
Tear lettuce into bite-size pieces and add all ingredients in large bowl. To serve, place in salad bowls and top with crumbled cheese and pine nuts.

Use olive oil and vinegar, vinaigrette, or any other dressing found in the recipe section.
Makes 6 to 8 servings

CARROTS PIQUANT

This recipe contains sesame and poppy seeds, both of which are rich sources of essential fatty acids. The carrots provide a significant amount of vitamin A (as beta carotene), and the turmeric serves as a top source of bioflavonoids. The garlic provides trace minerals, such as surfur, selenium, calcium, and germanium. Chili powder is very high in magnesium, and there is hardly a better source of potassium than coriander — and it tastes good!

1 lb. of carrots
2 teaspoons of fresh ginger, finely diced
4 cloves garlic, finely diced
¼ cup green onions, diced
4 teaspoons poppy seeds
2 teaspoons sesame seeds
½ teaspoon chili powder
½ teaspoon turmeric
1 teaspoon cumin
2 teaspoons ground coriander seeds
1 tablespoon sesame or olive oil

Wash carrots well and peel. Cut carrots in half through the width and slice into thin strips lengthwise. In a large non-stick skillet, saute' carrots and onions in oil until just tender. Remove carrot/onion mixture and set aside. Add ginger, garlic, poppy, and sesame seeds in skillet and stir over medium heat for 2 to 3 minutes. Add water if necessary. Stir in the rest of the ingredients including carrot/onion mixture, cook for an additional 3 to 4 minutes, and serve.
Makes 6 to 8 servings

BRUSSELS SPROUT SALAD WITH AVOCADO-VINAIGRETTE DRESSING

Brussels sprouts are an excellent, although under-used, food. They are both tasty and nutritious, being one of the richest vegetable sources of vitamin C. They are also an excellent source of potassium. Brussels sprouts are almost 90% water and contain only a few calories (only 50 calories per cup).

2 cups Brussels sprouts
1 carrot, shredded
1 grapefruit, peeled and sectioned (or use 1 cup diced cantaloupe or honeydew)
1/4 cup walnuts, chopped

DRESSING:

2 tablespoons vinegar
1 tablespoon avocado
1/2 teaspoon brown mustard
1/4 cup cold-pressed soy or sunflower oil

Salad: remove membranes from grapefruit and set aside. Wash sprouts and remove discolored outer leaves. Steam Brussels sprouts until tender and cool. Once cooled, slice the steamed sprouts using a sharp knife. Combine with carrot, grapefruit (or melon) and walnuts.

Dressing: add vinegar, mustard and avocado in blender or food processor, and blend till smooth. Gradually add oil while blending until mixture is thick.

Add enough dressing to moisten salad and toss. Reserve left-over dressing for other salads.
Makes 4 servings

BRUSSELS SPROUT-CARROT-CELERY SALAD

This makes a good, crunchy salad from winter vegetables. Carrots are added to increase the vitamin A value of the salad, since Brussels sprouts are only a moderately good source.

2 cups Brussels sprouts
1 cup chopped celery
1 cup carrots, diced
2 tablespoons walnuts (optional)

Wash sprouts and remove discolored outer leaves. Steam until tender and chill. With a sharp knife, thinly slice sprouts. Combine ingredients and toss with enough vinaigrette dressing to moisten. Add walnuts, if desired. Serve immediately.
Makes 6 servings

YOGURT-CUCUMBER SALAD

1 large, thin cucumber (or 2 medium-sized)*
1/4 teaspoon garlic powder (or 1 garlic clove, crushed)
1/2 teaspoon salt
1/2 teaspoon dry, crushed mint (or, 1 tablespoon fresh mint leaves, diced)
2 cups homemade or 2 small cartons yogurt (plain)**

Cut cucumber into quarters and slice. Add cucumber slices, garlic, pepper, salt, and mint; mix well. Mix in yogurt and serve.

SPINACH SALAD

2 lbs. spinach, chopped
2 cucumbers, sliced in half circles
1/2 cup fresh lemon juice (use vinegar if you have a citrus allergy)
3 garlic cloves, crushed
3 green or red peppers, sliced into strips
2 avocados, cubed
1/2 teaspoon onion powder.

Mix all ingredients in a large bowl. Refrigerate for three hours and serve.
Makes 6 servings

CAPER-ALMOND SALAD

butter lettuce (enough for 2 servings)
3 green onions, sliced
2 tablespoons almonds, slivered
capers
vinaigrette *or* olive oil and vinegar dressing
beet slices

Toss torn butter lettuce with green onions. Top with capers and slivered almonds. Garnish with beet slices.

 * Avoid fat cucumbers due to large seeds.
** This dish is much tastier if home-made yogurt is used.
Makes 4 servings

MEDITERRANEAN SALAD

1 large head of lettuce
4 leaves romaine lettuce
2 tomatoes, cubed
1/2 red sweet pepper, cut in strips
1/2 green pepper, cut in strips
2 cucumbers, peeled and sliced
1 stalk celery, sliced
3 stems green onions, sliced (optional)

DRESSING:

1/8 teaspoon black pepper
1 clove garlic, finely minced (or 1/8 teaspoon garlic powder)
1 tablespoon fresh or dried mint
1 teaspoon salt
juice of 1/2 lemon
2 tablespoons fresh parsley, finely chopped (or 1 tablespoon
  parsley flakes)
   Dressing: In a bottle, add olive oil, salt, lemon juice, mint, black pepper, garlic, and parsley. Tighten lid and shake well. Refrigerate overnight to blend flavors.

   Salad: Cut lettuce in half. Slice each half into strips and chop core into cubes. Wash in a strainer twice and let drain. Add the remainder of ingredients and refrigerate for at least 2 hours. When ready to serve, add dressing and eat immediately for the finest taste.
Makes 4 to 6 servings

CABBAGE SALAD WITH ONIONS

1 head cabbage, shredded
1/4 cup onion, shredded
1/2 teaspoon salt
1/4 teaspoon black pepper
1/2 lemon, squeezed
1/4 cup chopped parsley
pinch garlic salt (optional)

In a large salad bowl, add onion, salt, pepper, parsley and lemon juice. Mix well. Seasoning can be modified as desired.
Makes 8 servings

STEAMED CABBAGE SALAD VINAIGRETTE

4 cups finely shredded cabbage
2 tablespoons cold-pressed safflower, soy, or sunflower oil
1 tablespoon cider vinegar
1/4 teaspoon brown mustard
garlic salt to taste

Steam cabbage for 3 to 4 minutes, just until crisp-tender. Combine oil, vinegar, and mustard and pour over hot cabbage. Serve immediately or chilled.
Makes 6 to 8 servings

LEMON COLE SLAW

3/4 head green cabbage, grated
1/2 head purple cabbage, grated
2 large carrots, grated
3 stalks celery, chopped
1 cup green or red pepper, chopped

Mix the above together.

In a blender or food processor, mix:

juice of two lemons
1/2 tomato
1 clove garlic
1/4 cup olive oil
1 tablespoon dill weed
1 tablespoon caraway seed (optional)
1/2 teaspoon cumin (optional)

Blend until smooth and toss with cabbage salad.
Makes 6 servings

ARTICHOKE-AVOCADO SALAD

1 ripe avocado
1 small jar marinated artichokes
1/2 cup salsa or picante sauce
1/3 cup onion, chopped
1/2 cup radishes, sliced
2 tomatoes, diced
2 tablespoons olive oil
1/4 teaspoon pepper
salt to taste
lettuce

Drain artichokes and discard oil. Combine artichokes, picante sauce, onion, olive oil and radishes in a large mixing bowl. Add pepper and salt. Cover and chill for 2 to 3 hours. Add tomatoes. Cut avocado into strips and add. Serve on a bed of lettuce.
Makes 2 servings

VEGETABLE DISHES
GREEN BEANS IN OLIVE OIL

1 large onion, diced
6 cloves fresh garlic, grated (or 1 teaspoon of garlic powder)
1 large tomato, cubed
2 lbs. fresh or frozen green beans
1/2 cup olive oil
1/4 cup fresh parsley (or 2 teaspoons parsley flakes)
1/2 teaspoon black pepper
1 tablespoon salt
1/2 teaspoon lemon pepper
1/4 cup lemon juice.

If using fresh green beans, remove stems and cut into 2-inch pieces; set aside. Heat oil in a large frying pan for one minute; add onions. Cook for 2 to 3 minutes or until tender. Add tomatoes, green beans, black pepper, parsley, lemon juice, salt, and lemon pepper. Stir for one minute and cover. Cook for 25 to 30 minutes on medium heat. Serve immediately.
Makes 8 to 10 servings

RED CABBAGE CURRY

1 tablespoon olive oil
2 teaspoons mustard seeds
1 teaspoon curry powder or turmeric
1 small red onion, quartered and sliced thin
1 small head red cabbage, thin sliced
2 tablespoons lemon or lime juice, fresh squeezed
1/2 teaspoon salt

In a large skillet, heat oil. Add spices and mustard seeds; simmer for a short time. Add onion and simmer for several minutes, stirring often. Add cabbage and salt. Mix and cook until cabbage begins to wilt. Add lemon or lime juice and serve hot.
Makes 4 servings

WALNUT/PINE NUT STUFFED ONIONS

4 medium Spanish or red onions
1/2 cup pine nuts
1/4 cup celery, chopped
2 tablespoons fresh parsley, minced
2 tablespoons walnuts, chopped
2 tablespoons green or red bell pepper, diced (optional)
1 teaspoon tarragon
1/2 teaspoon coriander

Bake onions in their skins in a preheated oven at 350 degrees for 25 to 30 minutes. Cut off tops and scoop out most of the insides, leaving 2 or three layers of onion plus the skin. Set aside scooped onion. Take a thin slice off the bottom (root end), being careful not to cut into the cavity so that the onion will stand upright.

Chop the set aside onion centers and in a medium bowl, add to the remaining ingredients. Stuff onion shells and place in oven for 25 to 30 minutes or until onions are tender.
Makes 4 servings

SIMPLE BAKED ONIONS

Onions are an excellent food choice. If you love them, do not hesitate to eat some every day. Onions stimulate digestion, improve circulation and are a wonderful energizer. They also help protect against the number one and two diseases — heart disease and cancer. Use them as an addition to entrees as often as possible.

2 large yellow or red onions

In a preheated oven at 350 degrees, bake onions in their skins for 30 to 40 minutes or until tender. Serve as is, and let each person cut into their own juicy onion.
Makes 2 servings

SAUTEED BEET GREENS

Beet greens, also known as beet tops, are a fine source of beta carotene, and also contain significant amounts of potassium, calcium, magnesium, iron, and vitamin C. They are also an excellent source of fiber. This recipe will work well for other greens, such as spinach, turnip tops, or mustard greens.

1 large bunch beet greens
2 tablespoons lemon juice, fresh squeezed
1 medium onion, coarsely chopped
2 cloves garlic, crushed
1/4 cup olive oil
1/4 teaspoon salt
1/8 teaspoon black pepper

In a wok or an extra large, deep skillet, add olive oil and onions, but do not heat. Dice stems of beet greens and beet leaves into bite-sized pieces. In a bowl, add lemon juice, salt, pepper, and garlic. Mix well. Heat oil on medium heat, and cook onions until limp but not brown. Add onions and garlic; saute' for 1 to 2 minutes. Add lemon juice, salt, and pepper; stir. Add leaves and stems; toss constantly using two spatulas. Cook until leaves turn bright green (about 2 to 3 minutes).
Makes 4 to 6 servings

SAUTEED COLLARD GREENS

Collards are a highly nutritious vegetable which originate from the cabbage family. In fact, collard greens may be regarded as a form of wild cabbage. This fact is important in understanding why collards are so nutritious. Unlike most vegetables available in the marketplace, collards have been changed very little by domestication. Collards, particularly the greens, are one of the richest vegetable sources of calcium. They are higher in protein than most vegetables and contain about the same amount of protein per serving as do grains — but without all the starch. One cup of stems and leaves provide nearly 100 mgs. of vitamin C, 2.4 mgs. of niacin, 10,000 I.U. of vitamin A, 468 mgs. of potassium, and 300 mgs. of calcium. So eat your heart's desire of collard greens — you will be well rewarded for it!

1 large bunch collard greens plus stems
1 large onion, coarsely chopped
4 cloves garlic, crushed
1 teaspoon salt
1/8 teaspoon pepper
3 tablespoons lemon juice, fresh squeezed (or 3 tablespoons vinegar, if you are allergic to lemon)
1/4 cup olive oil

Wash collards well in water. Cut stems from leaves, and slice leaves in half. Chop collard leaves and stems into bite-sized pieces and set aside. In an extra-large non-stick skillet or a wok, heat oil on medium heat; add onions, garlic and saute' for 1 to 2 minutes. Add lemon juice, salt and pepper and stir. Add leaves and stems, and toss constantly using two spatulas. Cook until leaves turn bright green (about 2 to 3 minutes). *Makes 4 to 6 servings)*

SQUASH STIR-FRY

This recipe offers the advantage of having several types of squash, as well as a number of other vegetables, thus increasing the quantity and variety of nutrients available. Yellow squash is a rich source of vitamin A. Zucchini is a good source of calcium and phosphorus. Red sweet peppers are very high in vitamins A and C. Onions provide high amounts of sulfur which is needed for healthy skin, hair and nails. They also contain a subtance known as *adenosine*, which helps in the production of cellular energy. Squash is 90-95% water and this is the reason why it becomes so soft when cooked.

2 tablespoons butter
1 large zucchini, sliced thin
1 medium red onion, diced
1 sweet red or yellow pepper, diced
4 medium-size yellow squash, sliced thin
3 tomatoes, peeled and quartered
1/8 teaspoon garlic salt
dash of pepper
1 cup Parmesan, or 2/3 cup grated goat's cheddar cheese (optional)

Melt butter in wok or large, heavy skillet but be careful not to burn. Add onion and pepper; stir for a few seconds. Add zucchini and yellow squash and cook until crisp-tender. Add tomatoes, salt, and pepper and stir well. If desired, sprinkle cheese over vegetables and toss gently until cheese melts.
Makes 8 servings

ZUCCHINI IN OLIVE OIL

3 medium-sized zucchini, cubed
2 medium tomatoes, cubed
1 medium onion, diced
2 cloves garlic, crushed
1/4 cup olive oil
1/4 teaspoon black pepper
1/2 teaspoon salt
1 tablespoon fresh parsley, chopped (or 1 tablespoon parsley flakes)
1/8 teaspoon dried or fresh basil

In a large frying pan, heat olive oil for 1 minute. Add onions and fry for two minutes, stirring constantly. Add salt, pepper, garlic, and tomatoes. Stir for one minute, adding zucchini, parsley, and basil. Stir occasionally for 15 minutes over medium-low heat. Serve hot.
Makes 4 servings

BLENDER GAZPACHO (Gazpacho Drink)

1/2 cup onion, chopped
3 tomatoes, quartered
2 cloves garlic, diced
1 medium green pepper, chopped
1 small cucumber, peeled and sliced
1 teaspoon salt
4 tablespoons lemon or lime juice
2 tablespoons olive oil
1/2 cup water
2 tablespoons picante sauce

Add all ingredients into blender or food processor. Blend until vegetables are finely chopped. Serve in chilled bowls or cups. You can make this into a gazpacho drink by thinning it with tomato or V-8 juice.
Makes 4 one-cup servings

MOLDED GAZPACHO

2 envelopes unflavored gelatin
1 cup water
1 lb. tomatoes
1/2 cup green pepper, chopped
1/2 cup onion, finely chopped
2 tablespoons parsley, chopped
2 tablespoons fresh lemon juice
2 tablespoons apple cider vinegar
1/8 teaspoon cayenne pepper
2 cloves garlic, crushed
salt to taste

Add gelatin to 1/3 cup water and soak. Bring other 2/3 cup to a boil. Add gelatin and stir well until dissolved. Let cool. Add remaining ingredients and refrigerate.
Makes 6 servings

SESAME-GARLIC TOMATOES

2 teaspoons sesame oil
1 teaspoon sesame seeds
1 clove garlic, minced
2 cups cherry tomatoes
1/3 medium onion, finely chopped
1/4 teaspoon coriander

Heat oil in skillet and add garlic and onions, stirring to keep them from scorching. Reduce heat and add tomatoes plus coriander; cook for 5 to 10 minutes, stirring occasionally. Serve hot and top with sesame seeds.
Makes 4 servings

ZUCCHINI CANOES

3 zucchini, whole
1/2 cup zucchini, chopped
1 cup celery, chopped
1 cup yellow squash, chopped
6 tomatoes, chopped

2 onions, chopped
3 garlic cloves, minced
1/2 block tofu, crumbled (optional)
1 medium red pepper, diced

Saute' in small amount of olive oil, one onion and tofu — set aside. Saute' second onion, red pepper and celery for 4 minutes. Add zucchini and yellow squash and cook for an additional 4 minutes. Season with salt and pepper if desired.

Cut zucchini in halves and scrape out center. Fill zucchini with vegetable mixture, sprinkle onion-tofu mix on top, and bake for 1/2 hour at 350 degrees. Eat hot or use as a nutritious snack.
Makes 6 servings

DILLED BROCCOLI/CAULIFLOWER COMBO

1/2 pound broccoli, fresh
1 medium-sized head of cauliflower
1/2 teaspoon lemon juice (preferably fresh)
1/2 teaspoon dill weed
1 tablespoon butter

Cook vegetables in small amount of water or steamer until tender but still crisp. Add lemon juice, dill, and melted butter and toss.
Makes 4 servings

GRILLED SQUASH MEDLEY

Squash is an excellent food choice, as it is high in nutrients and quite low in starch and calories. Some types of squash, such as winter squash, are an excellent source of vitamin A (beta carotene). The squash varieties in this recipe provide good quantities of calcium, magnesium, potassium, vitamin C, and beta carotene. For this recipe, select squash no more than 1-1/2 inch in diameter.

2 zucchini squash, whole
2 Japanese eggplant
2 small yellow squash
olive oil
garlic salt
pepper

Slice all squash and eggplant lengthwise. Brush with a little olive oil. Sprinkle garlic salt and pepper to taste. Grill over hot coals for 6 to 8 minutes on each side or until just tender.
Makes 6 servings

ROOTS AND SUCH STIR FRY

Root vegetables are some of the healthiest foods known to mankind. As the name implies, these vegetables draw nutrients directly from the soil. Thus, it is not surprising that root vegetables are extra-rich in certain trace minerals, such as selenium, magnesium, potassium, sulfur, germanium, silicon, etc. This medley of roots and vegetables provide an abundance of potassium, selenium, phosphorus, calcium, beta carotene, and vitamin C.

3 small turnips
4 medium carrots
1 small green pepper
1 small red pepper
1 small red onion
2 medium parsley roots (save tops)
8 mushrooms, fresh
1 small sweet potato (optional)
1/4 head red cabbage, finely shredded
1/4 cup olive oil
3 tablespoons Dr. Bronner's Mineral Bouillon Base (optional)

Chop coarsely all the above ingredients (except cabbage). Heat oil in skillet or wok until hot taking care not to allow oil to smoke. Add turnips, carrots, and peppers to oil, stirring constantly for 5 minutes. Add remaining ingredients and cook until slightly tender (about 2 minutes). Then add cabbage and Dr. Bronner's bouillon. Stir for one minute and serve immediately. For an entree, add 1 cup cubed chicken or turkey.

Note: Dr. Bronner's Bouillon contains blackstrap molasses (sugar calories) and the sweet potato contains a significant amount of starch calories. Although both are rich food sources of nutrients, for most people following this diet, it is safer to omit these from the recipe. They may be added at a later time, when tolerance for natural sugars and starches.
Makes 6 servings

PICKLED TURNIPS

Most people have never eaten turnips. If you try to purchase them at a grocery store, nine times out of ten the checker won't know what they are. This recipe offers a convenient and delicious way to get a weekly dose of turnips. There are only a few ways to make turnips into a tasty part of a cooked meal, so it is best to eat them raw. This recipe provides you with raw turnips which are both delicious and more digestible than they would be otherwise. The pickling process, using vinegar, garlic and spices, breaks the fibers of the turnip down, making it easier for the digestive mechanism to liberate the nutrients. Why eat turnips on a regular basis? Because they are one of the richest vegetable sources of selenium, provided they are grown in selenium-rich soil. They also contain significant amounts of vitamin C, calcium, and potassium.

Turnip greens are one of the most nutritious vegetables known. They may well be the richest vegetable source of vitamin A (beta carotene), containing over 15,000 I.U. per cup. In addition, they contain very high amounts of calcium, magnesium, potassium, phosphorus, iron, zinc, vitamin E, vitamin C, and folic acid.

When you finish all your pickled turnips and turnip greens, be sure to drink the juice. As you can imagine, it is loaded with nutrients.

6 to 10 medium-sized turnips
1/4 cup vinegar
2 to 3 teaspoons salt
3 cloves garlic, thinly sliced
1 quart-sized mason jar (with new lid)
1 medium beet
turnip leaves (a few)

Wash turnips, beet, and turnip leaves thoroughly. Peel turnips and cut into wedges. Add to jar. Peel beet and boil in small amount of water until it softens — save the juice. Cut beet into wedges. Add turnips, beet wedges and garlic to jar. Follow with salt, vinegar, and beet juice. Fill with water (must be boiled) if necessary. Stuff with turnip leaves and seal tightly. Once cured, use as a snack, or as a vegetable dish with meat entrees.

PICKLED RED AND GREEN PEPPERS

1 large red sweet pepper
1 large green pepper
1 small hot red pepper (optional)

3 cloves garlic, finely sliced
1/4 teaspoon pickling spice
1/4 cup vinegar
1 tablespoon salt
1 quart-sized mason jar with new lid

Wash peppers well. Core peppers, remove seeds, and cut into slices. Place pepper and garlic slices in jar. Add spices, vinegar, and hot pepper (if desired). Fill with water (must be boiled), and seal tightly. Once cured, use as a snack or with entrees.

FRUIT DISHES

GRAPEFRUIT MEDLEY

The idea of combining grapefruit with vegetables originated in Guatemala. When properly combined, fruits and vegetables can be very tasty, as this recipe demonstrates.

3 large grapefruits
1 small sweet red bell pepper, cored and diced
2 teaspoons fresh onion, minced
2 tablespoons fresh parsley, minced
1/2 teaspoon red pepper (hot), crushed
1/2 teaspoon salt

With a serrated knife, peel the grapefruits taking care to remove all the white outer lining. Cut the membranes and take out the inner grapefruit segments, discarding the membranes. Cut the segments in halves or thirds and place in 2-quart bowl. Add remaining ingredients and mix gently. Refrigerate for at least 1 hour before serving.
Makes 6 to 8 servings

LOW-CARB FRUIT PLATTER

Certain fruits are relatively low in carbohydrates and, thus, are not fattening. Even the weight-conscious individual can relish in this fruitful delight. The fruits found on this plate contain 10% or less sugar.

1 cantaloupe, cut in halves
1/2 honeydew melon

1 papaya, peeled
1 pint strawberries, tops removed
parsley and sweet red pepper slices (as a garnish)

Always wash fruit carefully before preparing. Peel melons and cut into long slices 1-inch wide. Cut papaya into 1-inch cubes. Cut strawberries into halves. Arrange fruits on a large platters and garnish with parsley and red pepper slices.
Makes 4 to 6 servings

DICED FRUIT IN A BOWL

8-10 strawberries
1/2 cantaloupe
1 kiwi fruit
1 large wedge watermelon or honeydew melon

Wash all fruit well. Cut tops off of strawberries and slice in half. Remove peel from cantaloupe and dice into cubes 1/2-inch long. Peel kiwi and slice. Dice watermelon or honeydew melon into cubes 1/2 inch long. Gently mix fruit until uniformly blended. Chill and serve.
Makes 2 to 4 servings

FRUIT 'N NUT SALAD

1/2 honeydew melon
1/2 cantaloupe
1 large wedge watermelon
1/2 grapefruit, peeled
1 kiwi fruit
15-20 strawberries
1 whole papaya
1 whole guava (optional)
3 tablespoons pecans, chopped
3 tablespoons walnuts, chopped
1 tablespoon coconut, shredded (unsweetened)
2 one-half pint containers of real whipping cream (optional)

Make melons into melon balls. Take grapefruit sections and remove membranes. Peel kiwi fruit, and slice. Cut these slices in half. Cut strawberries in half. Peel papaya and guava and cut into segments. Add all fruit to a large bowl and mix gently. Top with pecans, walnuts, and coconut. If desired, use whipping cream as a topping. Pour whipping cream into bowl and whip with a hand or regular mixer.

DRINKS and SMOOTHIES

ENERGY SHAKE*

This high-protein shake provides a boost of energy for several reasons. First, both wheat germ and rice bran oil are rich, natural sources of vitamin E. Second, both oils contain special substances known to increase energy and stamina. Third, lecithin is an energizer. Fourth, the protein will help sustain energy levels by preventing blood sugar levels from falling. Last, but not least, the sugars in the honey, juice and/or fruit provide an easily digested, rapidly absorbed source of fuel for the body.

8 to 10 oz. water or juice
1 tablespoon wheat germ or rice bran oil
1 tablespoon lecithin granules
3 heaping tablespoons protein powder
2 tablespoons raw honey (optional)
Added fruit (unsweetened strawberries, blueberries, one-half banana)

Mix in blender and drink as a breakfast or between meal energizer.

PROTEIN DRINK

10 oz. water or juice
2-3 heaping tablespoons protein powder (unsweetened or sweetened with fructose only)
1 tablespoon of rice bran or Brewer's yeast (optional)

*This nutritious drink is not included on the first 90 days of the reduced carbohydrate diet.
Makes 1 large serving

Mix in blender or shaker and use as a between meal snack.
Makes 1 large serving

STRAWBERRY-ALMOND COOLER

1 pint fresh, ripe, strawberries
12 oz. almond milk, chilled

Add strawberries and almond milk to blender. Blend until smooth and serve.
Makes 2 servings

STRAWBERRY-GUAVA PUNCH

This drink will give you a punch in more ways than one. It is delicious and nutritious. For the weight conscious, it is low in sugar. For anyone with fatigue, it is the perfect booster — you can add some protein powder for an extra lift. Guavas are a rich source of vitamin C, and between these two fruits plus the lemon, you get over 200 mgs. of vitamin C per 10 oz. serving.

12 to 15 fresh, chilled strawberries
1 guava
2 tablespoons fresh-squeezed lemon or lime juice (optional)
20 oz. sparkling mineral water

Wash strawberries and remove tops. Add all ingredients to blender or juicer. Alter amount of water as desired. Serve immediately. Any remainder should be consumed within 48 hours since vitamin losses increase with time.
Makes 4 servings

CRANBERRY JUICE CREAMY SURPRISE

Pure, unsweetened cranberry juice is good for the body. Cranberries are an excellent source of bioflavonoids and a fair source of vitamin C as well as potassium. Of particular importance is the fact that cranberries contain a special bioflavonoid known as *anthocyanin*, the substance responsible for their brilliant red color. Researchers have found that anthocyanin inhibits the formation of tumors. This colorful substance exerts another remarkable action—it aids in restoring vision and helps improve the ability of the eyes to adapt from light to dark.

Cranberries are naturally low in sugar and so is pure cranberry juice. This presents a slight problem — it is so sour that few could drink it by itself. This recipe solves this problem with the addition of ripe honeydew melon, one of the most naturally sweet of all fruits. The key to the success of this recipe is to use the inner lining (the mushy part) of the melon, and to pour in any melon juice in the core.

1 large chilled, ripe honeydew melon
½ cup pure, unsweetened cranberry juice*

Cut melon in half and remove seeds, being careful to retain any juice. Scrape inner, mushy part of melon and measure two cups; place in blender and add any melon juice plus cranberry juice. Blend until smooth and serve. *Makes 2 servings*

CHLORELLA COOLER

The health benefits of chlorella are many. A single-cell algae, chlorella is one of the oldest known plants on this earth, dating back more than 2.5 billion years. Obviously, it is a very hardy creature. Chlorella contains more chlorophyll than any other known plant, and chlorophyll is nature's detoxifier. Chlorella contains a substance known as *chlorella growth factor,* which helps soothe and heal damaged tissue. This substance is of tremendous value in healing the lining of the intestines. Conditions for which chlorella has been found useful include:

acne
bladder infections
cancer
growth failure
lead poisoning
memory loss

allergies
cadmium poisoning
diabetes
halitosis (bad breath)
liver disease
pesticide & herbicide
poisoning

Chlorella has the unique attribute of being one of the oldest known forms of life still in existence, being nearly as old as the earth itself. Today, everyone can benefit from this wonderful substance. Although its taste is pleasant, most Americans have never tried algae as an edible substance. This recipe increases chlorella's palatability and makes it convenient to take on a regular basis.

*An excellent unsweetened cranberry juice is made by Lakewood Products of Miami, Florida and can be found in most health-food stores.

1 packet chlorella granules (see appendix B)
6 to 8 fresh strawberries, chilled
10 oz. chilled water
2 or 3 ice cubes

Stir chlorella into chilled water. Add all ingredients to blender and blend. Serve cold. A good rule of thumb is to drink at least 2 chlorella coolers per week.
Makes 1 serving

CARROT AND CREAM COOLER

This drink is both filling and nutritious. It is excellent as a refreshing drink on a hot day or as an addition to a meal. One serving of carrot juice provides the minimum daily requirement of vitamin A. The almond milk provides protein and minerals such as potassium and magnesium. This drink is far superior to any beverage you could buy in the grocery store, not to speak of nutrient-free drinks like pop, Kool-Aid, fruit drinks, and alcohol.

5 oz. carrot juice, chilled (preferably fresh-squeezed or canned)
5 oz. almond milk, chilled*

Mix in blender or by hand and serve.
Makes 2 servings

Note: This is an excellent drink for the person with blood sugar problems. Carrot juice should be used as a drink at a frequency no greater than every other day. Be sure to use it within 48 hours, since beta carotene oxidizes once exposed to air.

APRICOTS AND CREAM DELIGHT

Apricots are another very rich source of beta carotene, and they are relatively low in sugar. What makes them fattening is all that sugar added to the apricot products which are found at the supermarket. Check your health food store to see if unsweetened apricot products are available.

*Unsweetened almond milk may be difficult to find. Fresh almond milk can be made from blanched almonds. In a blender simply add 1/2 cup blanched almonds to 2 cups cold water and run at high speed for 3 minutes. Strain if necessary.

4 oz. unsweetened chilled apricot juice or puree — dilute with water if too thick

6 oz. almond or other nut milk, chilled

Add all ingredients in blender, mix for a few seconds, and serve.
Makes 2 servings

TROPICAL FRUIT N' CREAM

Some tropical fruits are low enough in sugar to be used on this program, such as fresh papaya. Papaya is a digestive stimulant, since it contains enzymes which assist digestive processes. Papayas also contain a significant amount of potassium, vitamin A, and vitamin C. Coconut milk is not just for taste. It too contains valuable nutrients, such as potassium, phosphorus, and calcium. Almonds provide the much needed mineral magnesium, being one of the richest natural sources of this important nutrient.

1/4 cup chilled coconut milk, fresh or canned*
1 cup almond or other nut milk (chilled)
1 whole papaya, peeled and diced
water (as needed)

Cut papaya into slices and set aside. Put nut milks in blender and blend at low speed. Add papaya, a few pieces at a time and blend until creamy. Add water or ice to change thickness. For another exciting flavor, add a few ripe strawberries.
Makes 2 servings

MELON SMOOTHIE (CANTALOUPE)

2 cups chilled cantaloupe, cut into cubes
3 ice cubes

Add ingredients to blender and blend until smooth. Serve garnished with mint leaves and a wedge of lemon or lime.
Makes 2 servings

* If canned coconut milk is used, it should be of the consistency of milk, but no thicker.

MELON SMOOTHIE (HONEYDEW)

1 whole honeydew melon
3 ice cubes

Wash outside of melon and slice in half. Scoop out seeds but save any juice. Remove outer peel and cube. Add melon, juice, and ice to blender and blend until smooth. Serve garnished with mint leaves and wedge of lemon or lime.
Makes 4 servings

WATERMELON SMOOTHIE

3 cups chilled watermelon, seeds removed
4 ice cubes

Place melon and ice cubes in blender; blend until smooth and serve.
Makes 2 servings

DRESSINGS, DIPS and SAUCES

VINAIGRETTE DRESSING

1/4 cup vinegar
2 large egg yolks
1/2 tablespoon salt
1 teaspoon pepper, freshly ground
2 cups olive oil or cold-pressed vegetable oil

Add 1/2 the oil and the rest of the ingredients to a food processor. Blend for 5 seconds. Transfer to a mixing bowl and gradually whisk in the rest of the oil. Add other spices if desired.

CARROT AND AVOCADO DRESSING

1 cup carrot juice
1 avocado, peeled
1 large red sweet pepper, cored and diced
2 tablespoons balsamic or apple cider vinegar
1/4 teaspoon salt

Place all ingredients in a blender or food processor and blend until smooth. Use as a dressing for salads or as a sauce or dip.

GUACAMOLE

1 large ripe avocado
1-1/2 tablespoons fresh lemon or lime juice
1/4 cup onion, minced
1 tablespoon diced green chili peppers
1/2 teaspoon garlic, minced
1/2 teaspoon cayenne pepper
1/2 teaspoon sea salt

Combine all ingredients in food processor or blender and process until smooth.

HUMMUS (GARBANZO BEAN DIP)

2 cans garbanzo beans (save 1/2 cup juice)
1/4 cup water
3 tablespoons tahini (sesame seed paste)
1 clove garlic
1/2 cup reconstituted lemon juice or 1/3 cup fresh lemon juice
2 tablespoons olive oil
parsley and paprika (for garnish)

Heat in a saucepan, garbanzo beans and water for 2 to 3 minutes or until hot. In a food processor, add beans, tahini, lemon, garlic, and salt. Mix until smooth (about 4 minutes). If too dry, add 1/4 cup of juice from beans. Serve in shallow bowl with olive oil poured on top. Sprinkle with paprika and chopped parsley.

GARLIC-DILL DRESSING

3 tablespoons lemon juice
2 tablespoons olive oil
1 teaspoon garlic salt
1 teaspoon dill seed
2 tablespoons fresh, minced parsley

Whip all ingredients in blender. Add water if necessary. Use as a salad dressing.

SUGARLESS MAYONNAISE

1/2 cup flax seed oil
1/2 cup olive or cold-pressed sunflower oil
1 egg, whole
2 tablespoons vinegar (may use lemon juice instead)
dash white or cayenne pepper

Mix oils together in a cup. In blender, break egg and add vinegar (or lemon juice), dash of pepper, and 1/4 cup of oil. Cover blender and blend at low speed. Just as it begins to thicken, add the remaining 3/4 cup of oil in a heavy stream while continuing to blend at low speed.
Makes 1-1/2 cups

SOYBEAN HUMMUS

This recipe is lower in carbohydrates than garbanzo bean dip and should be the "hummus of choice" during the first 90 days of the diet. Both, however, are excellent and healthy dishes. The soybeans and tahini paste provide essential fatty acids which are so desperately needed and difficult to get through the diet. Eat this dish as often as you can.

1 cup cooked soybeans
1/3 cup sesame tahini
1/2 cup lemon juice, freshly squeezed
3 tablespoons water
4 to 6 cloves garlic
1 tablespoon olive oil
1 teaspoon parsley and paprika (for garnish)

In a blender, add tahini, soybeans, lemon juice, water and garlic, and process on low speed until smooth. Chill and serve as a dip or sauce. Top with paprika and chopped parsley.

SUGAR-FREE TOMATO SAUCE

1 onion, chopped
1/2 cup celery, chopped
2/3 cup green pepper, chopped
2/3 cup carrots, chopped
1/4 cup fresh parsley, chopped
3 cloves garlic, diced

1 large can (1 lb.-12 oz.) whole, peeled tomatoes, pureed
2 large cans tomato sauce (unsweetened)
2 bay leaves
2 teaspoons oregano
1 teaspoon dried basil leaves
1/4 teaspoon pepper
1/2 teaspoon salt

In a large saucepan, saute' onions, vegetables, garlic and parsley in a small amount of olive oil for 4 minutes or until limp. Add remaining ingredients. Mix well. Bring to a boil then reduce heat. Keep uncovered and simmer for 30 minutes or until flavors blend. Freeze in small portions and use as needed.

HEARTY SALSA SAUCE

Salsa can be used as a sauce or dip. Spices may be tailored depending on how hot you like it. This salsa makes an excellent dip for sliced fresh vegetables or as a sauce over cooked vegetables.

One 4 oz. can green chili peppers, seeded and chopped
4 tomatoes, chopped
4 green onions, chopped
1 clove garlic, chopped
1 teaspoon oregano
1 tablespoon olive oil
1 teaspoon mustard seeds
juice of half a lemon
salt
pepper

Add all ingredients to a bowl and mix. Serve chilled or as is.

VEGETABLE DIP

2 cups vegetables (green beans, zucchini, carrots, broccoli, yellow squash, or cauliflower)
1 teaspoon minced onion
1 tablespoon minced green pepper
1 tablespoon vegetable seasoning
1/4 teaspoon dried dill weed (or 1/2 teaspoon fresh dill weed)
1/8 teaspoon sea salt

Cook vegetables in a steamer for about 5 minutes. Let cool. Blend on high speed and add onion, peppers, dill weed, salt, and seasoning. Serve with fresh vegetables as a dip.

EGGPLANT DIP

1 large eggplant
1/2 cup yogurt (if milk-sensitive, use 1/2 cup diced avocado)
1 clove garlic, crushed
1 tablespoon olive oil
1 tablespoon fresh parsley, finely chopped
dash cayenne pepper
salt to taste

Cook whole eggplant under broiler or in oven until soft (400-450 degrees). Let cool and remove pulp, discarding skin. Place pulp in cheese cloth or kitchen linen and squeeze liquid out until eggplant is dry. Add together eggplant and remaining ingredients in a blender and blend until thoroughly combined. Chill and serve as a dip for vegetables and meats or as a side dish by itself.

CREAMY GARLIC-AVOCADO DRESSING

3 cloves garlic, minced
1-1/4 cups cottage cheese
1 medium avocado, peeled
2 tablespoons fresh parsley, chopped
2 teaspoons vinegar
1/2 teaspoon onion salt

Remove the outer green peel of the avocado and dice. Add all ingredients to food processor or blender and blend until smooth.

EXTRA-STRENGTH HORSERADISH DRESSING

Horseradish is good for you. It contains numerous enzymes (the reason for its biting taste), most notably, *peroxidase,* which is useful since it helps preserve tissues. Peroxidase is, in effect, a ***natural preservative*** for your cells. Recently, it has been shown that peroxidase and other enzymes can be absorbed through the intestines into the bloodstream to be used by the cells and organs. Eat horseradish as often as you like.

3 tablespoons lemon juice, fresh

1 tablespoon mustard

2 tablespoons horseradish

1/4 teaspoon black pepper

1 tablespoon parsley, freshly chopped

1 tablespoon minced garlic, or 1 clove fresh garlic

2 tablespoons fresh onion, minced or 1 teaspoon onion powder

Place all ingredients in a food processor or blender. Blend until smooth. Use as a dressing on salads, or as a dip for meats or vegetables. Spread on steaks and chops, this dressing will greatly add to their digestion.

FRESH TARRAGON DRESSING

4 teaspoons egg yolks (use fresh farm eggs, if possible)

4 tablespoons tarragon vinegar

4 tablespoons fresh, minced tarragon

1 cup cold-pressed sunflower, sesame, or walnut oil

dash pepper

dash salt

2 tablespoons fresh parsley, finely chopped

Combine all ingredients and one-half the oil in a food processor or blender and process until well mixed. While blending, slowly add the rest of the oil. Use as a dressing on salads or as a dip for vegetables.

BUTTERS and YOGURT
CLARIFIED BUTTER

Place one pound of pure, unsalted butter in heavy pan or skillet. Simmer until butter is completely melted. Let stand until white foamy froth forms on top of mixture. Carefully skim off foam and discard. This is the part of butter that burns. A clear golden liquid will remain. Use this for cooking and sauteing.

BETTER BUTTER

This recipe makes your butter richer in essential fatty acids, since flax seed oil is one of the richest natural sources. It also makes butter smoother and easier to spread.

1/2 cup butter
1/3 cup flax seed oil

Mix in blender at low speed until creamy. Use as a spread or in cooking.

HOME-MADE YOGURT

1 gallon whole milk
1/2 pint of whipping cream or 1 pint Half and Half
3/4 cup yogurt starter*

Use a 16-quart stainless steel pan. Rinse with cold water. Add milk and cream, then cover. Let boil on medium-high heat for 15 to 20 minutes. Stir every 5 minutes. CAUTION: Keep a constant eye on the milk during the last 10 minutes to avoid over-boiling. Keep pan lid ajar and let cool to lukewarm (approximately 2-1/2 hours). Add yogurt starter and mix well into milk. Cover and let stand 5 hours or overnight. Uncover and refrigerate 1 day. Your yogurt is now ready with active cultures. Eat plain and over meat dishes, salads, vegetables, or with fruits.

Makes 20 to 24 servings

GOAT'S MILK YOGURT

This recipe is especially valuable for those allergic to cow's milk. In this case, use powdered goat's milk, as its taste is not too overpowering.

7 cups water
3 cups goat's milk (preferably powdered)
starter culture or 2 to 3 acidophilus capsules

*Try to get an active bacterial culture from a source other than store-bought yogurts, which have weak or diluted cultures. Many Europeans, Russians, Turks, Armenians, and Middle Easterners have starter yogurt cultures which they use to make future batches. If you know someone who has access to a starter culture, I suggest this as the first choice. You can also use kefir milk as a starter. Always save a cup or two of your batch to use as a starter for the next one. Your second choice would be acidophilus cultures found in health-food stores. Use 3 to 4 capsules per batch.

Bring water to a boil in stainless steel pot. Let cool to about 100 degrees (just hot enough to touch without getting burned). Add acidophilus culture and cover, letting stand for 8 to 9 hours. Refrigerate and serve as needed. Be sure to save some starter for the next batch. When making yogurt, try to use water which is not chlorinated, since chlorine kills the acidophilus bacteria.

2. SPECIAL REMEDIES FOR SPECIFIC AILMENTS

COLDS OR FLU

1. *Avoid* eating solid foods, meats or starches.

2. *Eat* mainly fresh fruits and vegetables.

3. *Have* several bowls of homemade chicken soup. Try the Chicken "Cure A Cold" soup recipe.

4. *Take* raw honey (uncooked and unfiltered), 1/3 cup three to four times daily.

    Note: This remedy really works well. Pure honey contains many anti-infective agents which boost immune power. The natural sugar helps fuel white blood cell into action against the virus or bacteria.

5. *Gargle* with salt water or preferably vinegar, 3 to 4 times daily.

6. *Sniff* water into your nostrils 3 to 4 times daily. Let the water drip back into the sinuses, then gently blow it out.

7. *Limit* your calorie intake (the old 7-Up and saltines remedy is out).

8. *Avoid* excessive nose blowing as this can drive the infection deeper into the sinuses, lungs, eardrum, or even into the brain.

9. *Take* liquid garlic extract, 5 capsules three times daily (see appendix B).

10. *Be sure* to take plenty of vitamin C and vitamin A. Recommended dosages would be 2 to 4 grams of vitamin C and 30,000 to 50,000 I.U. of vitamin A. Stay on this dosage for the duration of the illness only.

COLD SORES*

1. *Apply* aloe vera (straight from the plant or as a gel) to affected area.

*If cold sores are frequent, check for food allergies.

2. *Drink* aloe vera juice, at least 6 oz. daily.

3. *Take* large doses of vitamin C and bioflavonoids. Bioflavonoids are powerful in destroying the cold-sore virus. Take 2 to 4 grams of each daily until the lesions clear.

4. *Avoid* foods high in arginine (an amino acid). This includes all nuts and seeds, cocoa, and beans.

5. *Consume* foods rich in lysine, including cheese, milk, and meats.

6. *Take* extra lysine, 4 to 6 capsules per day.

7. *Try* bee pollen which has a high concentration of lysine.*

CONSTIPATION**

1. *Avoid* harsh laxatives.

2. *Eat* mainly fruits and vegetables.

3. *Start* your morning with 2 large glasses of warm water. Add to each either 1/2 cup fresh-squeezed lemon juice or vinegar.

4. *Drink* eight 10 oz. glasses of water daily. Constipation often indicates the existence of a mild state of dehydration.

5. *Take* 1/2 cup honey morning and night for at least three days **(caution: diabetics must omit this one).**

6. *Add* 1 to 3 heaping teaspoons of acidophilus culture three times a day mixed in water or juice.

7. *Try* some Sun Chlorella (loaded with chlorophyll) to help make the acidophilus grow.

Note: If the above are not sufficient, try four ounces of aloe vera juice three times per day (see appendix B).

*Lysine inhibits the growth of the cold-sore virus while arginine dramatically enhances its growth.

**For the grain-allergic individual there is no better cure than to remove the offending grains from the diet.

DIARRHEA*

1. *Rest* the digestive tract by fasting and by avoiding all meats and grains.

2. *Drink* lots of fluids, especially water and to a lesser degree, juices. The finest anti-diarrhea juices are peach, pear, and apricot.

3. *Avoid* citrus fruits or citrus juices as well as apple and grape juice.

4. *Eat* only fruits. Pureed vegetables are also allowed. Pure, home-made yogurt or kefir which are heavy in lactobacillus culture may benefit some. Drink the broth of homemade chicken soup.

5. *Take* honey, 1/3 cup 3 to 4 times daily. If diarrhea intensifies, up the dose to 1/2 cup four times daily

Note: For stubborn, persistent cases, you may try any number of nutritional medicines including *Tanalbit,* bentonite, or chlorella.**

INSOMNIA***

1. *Try* eating a snack right before bedrime. First try a high protein snack (cheese, eggs, sliced meat, nuts). If this doesn't work, try 1/3rd to 1/2 cup of honey in a warm glass of water or milk.

2. *Take* Calcium, 1000 to 2000 mgs. one half-hour before bedtime. If you awaken, take another dose.

3. *Add* 100 mgs. of niacin, 500 mgs. of pantothenic acid, and 100 to 500 mgs. of B-6 if the above isn't sufficient.

*persistent diarrhea in a child usually indicates intestinal parasites.

**Tanalbit is made by Scientific Consulting Services. It helps make the stools more solid (see appendix B).

***Stress, worry, and aggravation are major factors in causing insomnia, although food allergies and hypoglycemia are often related.

FOR WOMEN ONLY

MENSTRUAL CRAMPS

1. *Try* bromelain (uncoated), 3 to 4 tablets every four hours.*

2. *Avoid* sugar as it aggravates the cramps.

3. *Take* 2000 mgs. of calcium and 1000 mgs. of magnesium 2 to 3 days prior to and also during the cramping. These minerals sedate the pelvic nerves.

4. *Realize* that most women with severe menstrual cramps are deficient in several B-vitamins. Large doses of all of them are indicated. An excellent B-complex formula is manufactured by Cardiovascular Research (see appendix B).

5. *Add* fish oils and vitamin E if the above is not effective. Both help ease spasms and sooth inflammation.

Note: An infection within the female organs by yeasts or other organisms may either cause or aggravate menstrual difficulties. Often, cramps will be worse when these infections are active.

Thyroid malfunction is also a common cause of menstrual problems. Your thyroid function may need to be evaluated. Nutritional deficiencies impair its function. In such cases, routine blood tests for thyroid hormones are seldom abnormal.

* Bromelain is an enzyme which occurs naturally in the stem of pineapples. It is effective in reducing inflammation and improving circulation within the pelvic organs as well as throughout the body. Most bromelain tablets available in health food stores contain an enteric coating to protect the enzyme from destruction by stomach acid. Unfortunately, this coating often interferes with the absorption of the enzyme. For this reason, I recommend bromelain products which are *not* coated. An excellent and well-priced *uncoated* bromelain is made by GY&N products. This bromelain has a high potency and is well absorbed.

To order: GY&N PRODUCTS
c/o Nutritional Supplement Services
212 Willow Parkway
Buffalo Grove, Illinois 60089
1-800-243-5242

NAUSEA (INCLUDING NAUSEA OF PREGNANCY)*

1. *Try* ginger root, whole or ground, or as a tea. Take several times during the day.

2. *Avoid* solid foods until nausea clears.

3. *Take* 1000 to 1500 mgs. of calcium carbonate, a natural way to absorb excess acid.

4. *Eat* brown rice or rice bran as a source of thiamine and other B-vitamins.

5. *Add* beet juice crystals and B-complex vitamins if the above is not sufficient.

6. *Avoid* heavy meals, eating 5 to 6 small meals instead.

VAGINAL DISCHARGE

1. *Realize* that the most likely cause is yeast infection no matter what the doctors say. The second most likely cause is chronic infection from bacteria or parasites, such as trichomonas.

2. *Reduce* or eliminate your intake of sugar and starch.

3. *Rub* tea tree oil into the vaginal tract, morning and night. Dilute the tea tree oil with an equal part of olive oil, and apply directly to the vaginal walls. This is more effective and a lot safer than antibiotics. Tea tree oil is available in many health food stores, or by mail order:

NUTRITIONAL SUPPLEMENT SERVICES
212 Willow Parkway
Buffalo Grove, Illinois 60089
1-800-243-5242

4. *Cut out* all caffeinated beverages.

5. *Increase* your intake of garlic and onions which are especially helpful if they are raw or lightly cooked.

*Nausea can be a serious symptom. If it persists, check with your doctor.

6. *Take* a garlic supplement. The most effective type for directly killing yeasts and parasites is one made from uncooked garlic. One of the more effective garlic products for this purpose is known as Herbal Garlic, made by the Multiway Corporation. This item is available at Nutritional Consulting Services (see #3 above). The suggested dose is 1 capsule three times daily, to be increased within a week to 3 capsules three times daily.

7. *Include* an acidophilus/bifidus supplement, taking a dose morning and night daily. Do this regularly over the long term for best results.

8. *Inject* aloe Skin Balm through an applicator morning and night (see appendix B).

FOR MEN ONLY

PROSTATE TROUBLE

1. *Take* zinc, 50 to 150 mgs. per day. Once symptoms are improved, reduce the dosage to 25 to 50 mgs. daily.

2. *Flush* your prostate gland and urinary tract with large amounts of water.

3. *Heal* your prostate and urinary tract with chlorophyll. Rich sources of chlorophyll include chlorella, alfalfa, dark green vegetables, and chlorphyll extracts.

4. *Eat* a large handful of pumpkin or squash seeds two or three times daily.

5. *Add* 2 tablespoons of flax or sesame seed oil, morning and night.

6. *Try* bee pollen, one teaspoonful or 4 capsules three times daily. Ground bee pollen is preferable to whole pollen grains.

IMPOTENCE

1. *Eliminate* alcohol, since it causes impotence. Alcohol, if consumed regularly, causes atrophy of the testicles and reduces circulation to the sexual organs.

2. *Increase* your dosage of zinc. You can take between 75 to 150 mgs. per day, but once sexual function returns, reduce the dose.*

3. *Take* bee pollen, since it contains amino acids and hormones which stimulate sex drive. You need to stay on it for at least 4 months.

* Do not take large doses of zinc for prolonged periods unless you also take supplemental copper. Zinc in high doses interferes with copper absorption.

4. *Take* yohimbe root, a special herb proven to restore male sexual functions. Studies show that it helps in nearly half the cases.

5. *Add* Siberian ginseng, since it stimulates the activity of the sexual glands and increases circulation.

6. *Be sure* to increase your dose of selenium. Take at least 600 mcg. per day.

7. *Extra doses* of B-vitamins should be taken, as they assist all the functions related to the sexual glands.

8. *Vitamin E* helps improve circulation to the genitals and increases virility if taken in doses of 800-1600 I.U. per day.

RECEDING HAIRLINE

In many individuals, it is possible to stop the hair loss associated with male pattern baldness. In some instances, new hair growth can be stimulated. There are so many hair treatments, potions, and/or nutritional supplements available for treating this condition that figuring out what approach to take is often difficult. The following protocol will help guide you through this confusion. After several years of trial and error, these are the nutritional agents and lifestyle changes I have found to be most effective:

1. *Stop* the intake of alcohol if you are a drinker, and if you are a smoker, quit.

2. *Control* your stress, and if you are a worrier, reduce or stop the worrying. Both cause the muscles in the scalp to tighten, cutting off blood flow to the hair follicles.

3. *Use* a shampoo containing pure herbal extracts. Probably the finest is *Shampure*, which is made by the Aveda Corporation. Shampure also contains sources of essential fatty acids such as avocado oil. This oil is valuable for promoting strong, healthy hair shafts.

4. *Take* large amounts of essential fatty acids. The more the better. It is necessary to take extra vitamin B-6 to help in metabolizing the fatty acids. You'll need lecithin, primrose oil, cold pressed vegetable oil, and/or flax seed oil. The best thing to do is make a fatty acid cocktail and take it morning and night.

5. *Increase* your dosage of zinc to at least 100 mgs. per day. White spots on the nails indicate a severe zinc deficiency. This may indicate the need to take even higher doses of zinc. Do not exceed 150 mgs. per day.

6. *Try* the Medi-Plex hair loss regimen. This is the newest, most promising breakthrough in hair treatment. Clinical tests at independent labs have shown that regular use of Medi-Plex leads to an

enlargement in the diameter of hair shafts and also increases the number of hairs. Active ingredients include unique herbs and fatty acids which stimulate inactive hair follicles and keep active ones from degenerating. The result is improved hair growth, sheen, texture, and thickness. For more information about a doctor or center near you offering this program, contact:

MEDI-PLEX
2730 Wilshire Blvd., Suite 301
Santa Monica, California 90403
(800) 292-6006

7. *Take* a multiple vitamin which contains biotin, inositol, and silicon. These nutrients are often severely deficient in people with hair loss.

8. *Increase* your protein intake. Try one of the protein shakes listed in the recipe section. Be sure to take the protein regularly, at least twice per day.

9. *Kill* the fungus that is probably growing on your scalp. It is growing for sure if you have seborrhea or psoriasis of the scalp. Use *Balancing Infusion*, an oil-based solution, on the scalp at least twice per day. Rub the oils liberally into the scalp at night before bedtime. This, in my experience, is the most important step. By killing the fungus, you can stimulate new hair growth. Also, the oils and vitamins contained within this product nourish the hair follicles. This means that existing hair shafts become stronger, which prevents further hair loss. Balancing Infusion, as well as Shampure, can be ordered by contacting:

NUTRITIONAL SUPPLEMENT SERVICES
212 Willow Parkway
Buffalo Grove, Illinois 60089
1-800-243-5242

3. MAINTENANCE NUTRITIONAL SUPPLEMENT PROGRAM

I highly recommend that anyone who is concerned about his/her health take nutritional supplements. Ideally, it is best to undergo some testing first to see exactly what your deficiencies are. Fortunately, specialized tests are now available for detecting nutritional deficiencies within the cells. Only a few labs across the country perform these tests. The one I recommend is Nutritional Testing Laboratories, since they specialize in tests for nutritional and dietary imbalances. For more information contact:

NUTRITIONAL SUPPLEMENT SERVICES
212 Willow Parkway
Buffalo Grove, Illinois 60089
1-800-243-5242

Other tests may be of value, such as a hair analysis. Even a routine blood chemistry profile can provide signals of nutritional imbalances, provided the doctor is skilled at interpreting them (see Part III of the book, Section 2). Knowing that it is not always possible to get these tests, I have designed a maintenance program based upon the deficiencies seen in the majority of patients:

SUPPLEMENTS	DOSAGE
Multiple Vitamin/Mineral (without iron if you are a non-anemic male or post-menopausal female)	1-2 tabs or caps daily
B-complex	1-2 tabs or caps daily
Chlorella	15-30 small pills daily (optional)
Beta Carotene	25,000 I.U. daily
Vitamin E (as free tocopherols)	800-1600 I.U. daily
Selenium	300-600 micrograms daily, the higher dose being applicable in regions with selenium-deficient soil.*
Essential Fatty Acids (either as flax seed or primrose oil)	Tablespoon or 6 capsules daily
Cod Liver Oil** (or) Fish Oils (EPA/DHA)	Teaspoon daily or 8 capsules daily
Garlic (either as an oil, powder, or liquid extract)	6 capsules daily
Vitamin C	2-4 grams daily
Zinc	30-50 mgs. daily

*People living in regions with selenium-rich soil who eat plenty of fresh vegetables and meats from that locality may not need to take supplemental selenium.

**Cod liver oil offers the added benefit of being an excellent, natural source of vitamin A. Fish oil tablets contain little if any vitamin A.

This program gives you excellent protection against the ravages of modern living—pollution, radiation, toxic wastes, ozone, and heavy metals. You may have deficiencies of other nutrients than those mentioned. If you can find a nutritionally-oriented health practitioner, he might be able to discover these deficiencies.

Individuals who are exposed to even greater amounts of radiation or toxic chemcials need to double or even triple the dose of certain nutrients particularly garlic, beta carotene, chlorella, vitamin E, selenium, and vitamin C. A partial list of susceptible individuals includes:

artists	workers in chemical plants
auto mechanics	airline pilots
x-ray technicians	flight attendants
radiologists	frequent flyers
scientists	computer operators
painters	machinists
printing press operators	

No sane airline pilot, flight attendant, or frequent flyer should go without his/her daily dose of beta carotene. For this group, I advise taking at least 50,000 I.U. daily. Nor should a radiologist go a day without extra vitamin E and selenium. Cancer is far more frequent in these speciality fields. Why take chances? I'd rather see you practice overkill, that is, taking antioxidants to an excess rather than skimping on the only substances known to prevent cancer. It is far more dangerous to take too little than to take too much.

PART III
For Doctor's Only

I. NUTRITIONAL PROTOCOLS FOR SELECTED DISEASES

Below are listed some of the major diseases seen in America today along with the nutrients most commonly used to treat them. To be sure, there are many other important nutrients, herbs, and remedies beside those mentioned.

You will note that the remedies for each condition have been divided into 1st and 2nd Priority, and that a third category, Foods and Herbs, has also been listed. Those found in 1st Priority are the nutrients which have been firmly established by scientific and clinical studies to have a powerful curative effect. Those nutrients listed as 2nd Priority are useful in improving the disease process and in preventing its progression, although they may or may not have been proven useful through scientific studies. The beneficial effect of some of the substances listed under the category Foods and Herbs has been determined through scientific research, while others are listed as a result of clinical experience.

ACNE

1st Priority

vitamin A
vitamin E
vitamin B-6 (especially in
    adolescent acne)

2nd Priority

thiamine
biotin
beta carotene
fiber

riboflavin
niacin
acidophilus
zinc
essential fatty acids

Note: Food allergies should be ruled out.

ALCOHOL ADDICTION

1st Priority	2nd Priority
niacin	selenium
vitamin C	vitamin A
thiamine	vitamin E
vitamin B-6	tyrosine
folic acid	pantothenic acid
vitamin B-12	calcium
magnesium	manganese
zinc	silicon
potassium	chromium
essential fatty acids	
glutamine (an amino acid)	

FOODS AND HERBS

rice bran	ground flax seed
watermelon	fermented milk products
silymarin	

Note: Many alcoholics are allergic to sugar and/or grains. They may also be allergic to yeasts. Have your doctor perform the Food Intolerance Test if you are an alcoholic aspiring towards abstinance.

ARTHRITIS

1st Priority	2nd Priority
vitamin C	folic acid
vitamin A	vitamin B-12
vitamin E	copper
niacin	manganese

vitamin B-6
essential fatty acids
fish oils
vitamin D
bioflavonoids
magnesium
calcium
zinc
selenium
potassium
pantothenic acid

PABA
thiamine
riboflavin

FOODS AND HERBS

chlorella (see appendix B)
onion
alfalfa
coriander leaf
grape vinegar (Dr. Bronner's)

garlic
whole goat's milk
kelp
raw honey
fresh black cherries

CANDIDA ALBICANS INFECTION*

1st Priority
essential fatty acids
selenium
zinc
vitamin A
magnesium
vitamin B-6
thiamine
biotin
folic acid
riboflavin

2nd Priority
vitamin B-12
calcium
vitamin E
beta carotene
bioflavonoids
digestive enzymes

*This infection is prevalent primarily because of the overuse of antibiotics.

FOODS AND HERBS

goldenseal root

garlic

Tanalbit (see appendix B)

pau d'arco

onion

PurAloe (see appendix B)

CIGARETTE ADDICTION

1st Priority

tyrosine

calcium

vitamin C

vitamin E

beta carotene

folic acid

vitamin B-12

thiamine

niacin

2nd Priority

magnesium

riboflavin

pantothenic acid

Note: Few smokers quit with just nutrition alone. There must first be a desire to quit. If you smoke, the programs outlined in this book will not work for you until you quit.

DIABETES

1st Priority

chromium

niacin

thiamine

2nd Priority

selenium

vitamin E

vitamin A

biotin
vitamin C
essential fatty acids
zinc
magnesium
vitamin B-6
manganese
fiber

carnitine
vitamin C
vitamin B-12
bioflavonoids
fish oils
coenzyme Q-10
potassium

FOODS AND HERBS

rice bran (rich in chromium and B-vitamins)
olive oil (helps prevent circulatory damage)
cucumber
turnips with greens
Jeruselum artichoke
alfalfa
garlic
onion

GLAUCOMA

1st Priority

vitamin C (preferably as fresh
    fruit, vegetables, or rose-hips
    extract)
bioflavonoids
vitamin B-6
folic acid
chromium
vitamin A
pantothenic acid

2nd Priority

selenium
zinc
choline

HEART DISEASE

1st Priority

niacin
chromium
vitamin E
fish oils
selenium
carnitine
magnesium

2nd Priority

copper
zinc
vitamin A
vitamin B-6
folic acid
essential fatty acids

taurine
calcium
potassium
manganese
thiamine
coenzyme Q-10

FOODS AND HERBS

garlic
hawthorn berries
kelp
rice bran (for its B-vitamin content)

olive oil
onions
ground flax seed
avocado

HIGH BLOOD PRESSURE

1st Priority

potassium
magnesium
calcium
essential fatty acids
niacin
vitamin E
fish oils

2nd Priority

selenium
vitamin B-6
lecithin
vitamin C
bioflavonoids

FOODS AND HERBS

fermented milk products (the calcium is easier to absorb due to the
   fermentation process)
cod liver oil
turnip or mustard greens
collards

HYPOGLYCEMIA

1st Priority

chromium
niacin
thiamine
manganese
vitamin B-6
pantothenic acid
lipoic acid

2nd Priority

digestive enzymes
vitamin C
vitamin A
tyrosine
fiber

FOODS AND HERBS

dessicated liver tablets, with or between meals
wild ginseng tablets taken between meals
chlorella tablets taken between meals
bee pollen
raw honey (can be used to bring the blood sugar up when it drops)
rice bran (rich in B-vitamins and chromium)

HYPOTHYROIDISM

1st Priority	2nd Priority
thiamine	selenium
riboflavin	vitamin E
niacin	vitamin C
vitamin B-6	magnesium
zinc	calcium
copper	
potassium	
iodine	
tyrosine	
essential fatty acids	
vitamin A	

FOODS AND HERBS

kelp and other iodine-rich sea vegetation
rice bran (due to its rich thiamine and niacin content)
ocean fish
seafood, particularly shrimp

INFERTILITY

1st Priority	2nd Priority
folic acid	vitamin B-6
vitamin B-12	niacin
vitamin A	bioflavonoids
vitamin E	amino acids
vitamin C	iodine
selenium	
zinc	
essential fatty acids	

FOODS AND HERBS

royal jelly
chlorella

bee pollen
ginseng extract

OSTEOPOROSIS

1st Priority

calcium
magnesium
zinc
manganese
silicon
vitamin A
vitamin D
vitamin C
essential fatty acids
amino acids

2nd Priority

copper
boron
vitamin B-12
folic acid
riboflavin
vitamin K

PARKINSON'S DISEASE

1st Priority

vitamin E
vitamin C
vitamin B-6
selenium
thiamine
tyrosine

2nd Priority

beta carotene
calcium
magnesium
folic acid
vitamin B-12
lecithin

FOODS AND HERBS

chlorella (due to its rich RNA content)
wheat germ oil (due to its rich vitamin E content)
ginseng
cayenne pepper (improves circulation)

STOMACH OR DUODENAL ULCER

1st Priority

fiber
vitamin C
bioflavonoids
vitamin A

2nd Priority

selenium
vitamin B-1

STOMACH OR DUODENAL ULCER

1st Priority
fiber
vitamin C
bioflavonoids
vitamin A
zinc
essential fatty acids
vitamin U*
folic acid
vitamin E

2nd Priority
selenium
vitamin B-1

FOODS AND HERBS

Wakasa (an extract of chlorella which helps heal the ulcer)**
fresh-squeezed cabbage or potato juice
PurAloe (see appendix B)
ground flax seed
ground alfalfa seed

*This is the name given to what is actually a variety of compounds found in raw cabbage or cabbage juice. Fresh-squeezed cabbage juice is one of the finest remedies for gastric or duodenal ulcer.

**Wakasa, made by YSK International, has been proven in scientific studies to help heal ulcers by causing the intestinal lining to regenerate. Its effectivity in gastric ulcers is nearly 100%, while duodenal ulcer response is 70% or greater (See appendix B).

PART III

II. Interpretation Guide for Routine Blood Chemistry

The following information will help doctors interpret routine blood chemistry in a nutritional manner. The lab figures are given either as milligrams per deciliter, or units per liter.

GLUCOSE... if high (above 105), a tendency towards the development of diabetes is possible. If fasting blood sugar consistently runs high, it is likely that a chromium deficiency exists. Adding chromium to the diet in the form of Brewer's yeast, chromium picolinate or glucose tolerance factor should bring the blood sugar down. High sugar readings are also seen when the adrenal glands fail to work properly (known as adrenal insufficiency, chronic adrenal failure, etc.).

Biotin and thiamine deficiency are frequent. Fat soluble thiamine can be added (Allithiamine, see appendix B). Both niacin and pyridoxine help stabilize blood sugar levels. Magnesium helps drive glucose into the cells, and this may also be deficient. Fiber intake should be increased.

GLUCOSE..... if low (below 70), hypoglycemic tendencies exist. Again, supplemental chromium and thiamine are indicated. A diet high

241

in protein and low in sweets is suggested. Niacin and pyridoxine will help stabilze blood sugar levels.

Low blood sugar indicates that the adrenal glands are malfunctioning and are unable to prevent blood sugar levels from dropping. Levels may dip as low as 40 on occasion. Such drops explain mood swings, agitation, depression, and fatigue.

If the above symptoms exist, a glucose tolerance test may be indicated. Also, check magnesium levels in red cells. Magnesium is needed to drive glucose into the cells. Many hypoglycemics are deficient in magnesium as well as zinc. If white spots on the fingernails exist, be sure to give zinc, 50 to 100 mgs. daily.

It is crucial that hypoglycemic patients snack 2 to 3 times a day in addition to eating three regular meals. Emphasize breakfast which should be high in protein, although fresh fruit is often well tolerated. Snacks must be free of refined sugars, malt, corn syrup, etc.

CREATININE. . . . if high (above 1.2) think of chronic renal insufficiency. Levels over 1.4 are usually indicative of chronic renal failure. The kidneys can regenerate and, thus, mild elevations in creatinine levels are not always a cause for alarm. However, steadily increasing creatinine levels should not be taken lightly. In males, consider stasis of urine due to a swollen, inflamed prostate. In females, particularly, consider chronic infection (chronic pyelonephritis), especially if there is a history of bladder and/or kidney infections. The kidneys can be a reservoir for a variety of microbes ranging from E. Coli to yeasts and tuberculosis. These microbes often cause chronic infections which cannot be diagnosed by routine urine cultures.

In cases involving swollen prostate glands, zinc plus essential fatty acids are often curative. The kidneys begin to degenerate in essential fatty acid and/or vitamin A deficiency. Try two tablespoons of flax (linseed) oil, one tablespoon of cod liver oil along with 800-1200 I.U. of vitamin E daily. Foods rich in potassium should be eaten regularly.

If chronic infection is suspected, do not give antibiotics alone. If an organism can be cultured, give antibiotics to which the organism is sensitive along with nutritional agents. In either case, use the following nutritional program:

1. chlorella — 30 to 60 tiny tabs daily (for its chlorophyll content)
2. liquid garlic extract — 6 capsules three times daily
3. potassium and magnesium citrate — 6 to 12 capsules daily
4. cod liver oil — 1 tablespoon three times daily. Take this dosage for the duration of treatment only.
5. vitamin E — 800 to 1600 I.U. daily
6. lactobacillus acidophilus/bifidus culture — teaspoon three times daily.

7. essential fatty acids (flax seed oil or cold-pressed sunflower, safflower, soy, or walnut oil) — 4 to 6 tablespoons daily.
8. watermelon — eat large quantities or squeeze into juice. If using juice, drink 10 ounces three times daily. It acts as a mild, natural diuretic.
9. fluids — drink a minimum of eight 10 oz. glasses of either water or juice, but avoid orange and grapefruit juices as they may irritate the kidney/bladder.
10. honey — consume at least 10 ounces of pure, raw honey. Honey helps by regulating fluid balance. The sugars within honey, once absorbed, increase the water content of blood by a powerful osmotic effect. This results in an increased rate of urine flow through the kidneys. To get this benefit, it is necessary to consume large quantities of it. Do not be concerned about the sugar content of the honey. Unless the patient has a severe yeast infection, is allergic to sugars, has diabetes, or is severely hypoglycemic, it is harmless.
11. juices — of special value are the ones rich in potassium which include apricot, tangerine, pomegranate, papaya, beet, and parsley. In addition, most of these juices are rich in vitamin A (beta carotene).

CREATININE....if low (below .7), think of protein deficiency or impaired protein digestion. Lowered levels are often seen in vegetarians. Reduced amounts of hydrochloric acid or impaired secretion of pancreatic enzymes must be considered. Thiamine and niacinamide both increase the secretion of hydrochloric acid and other digestive juices. Digestive enzymes, 2 to 3 tablets with meals, may improve protein assimilation. In addition, pyridoxine and zinc are required for adequate protein digestion to proceed. The synthesis of digestive enzymes within the pancreas is dependent upon adequate tissue levels of both of these nutrients. Tissue pyridoxine levels can be assessed with the erythrocyte glutamate pyruvate transaminase test (see page 253).

SODIUM....if high (above 144), think first of dehydration. Kidney disease is possible, especially if potassium levels are also elevated. Water softeners or tap water contaminated with sodium can be responsible. If the adrenal glands are producing excess amounts of cortical hormones, blood sodium levels can be elevated. Water high in sodium should be avoided, and salt consumption in foods reduced. High doses of vitamin C, pantothenic acid, thiamine, niacin, and vitamin A will relax the adrenal glands and help stop sodium retention.

SODIUM....if low (below 139), think first of adrenal cortical insufficiency. The adrenal glands secrete aldosterone, a hormone which conserves sodium. When this hormone is lacking, sodium is easily lost through the kidneys. Other causes include acute or chronic diarrhea and kidney disorders. Most often, in a person who is not acutely ill, low sodium means chronic adrenal failure. Symptoms such as fatigue, headaches, indigestion, cold extremities, and constipation may also be elicited. The adrenal glands secrete over 50 hormones. Thus, the presentation of a person with adrenal insufficiency may be varied and complex. Their symptoms are often vague. Yet they do fit a pattern. If the sodium stays persistently low, look for other evidence of adrenal failure such as pigmentation changes, vitiligo, eczema, thin hair, hair loss on the outer third of the legs, and crowding of the lower incisors. Other findings on routine blood chemistry may include mild eosinophilia (above 1.5%), lymphocytosis, reduced cholesterol and an elevated serum potassium. If you suspect adrenal insufficiency, a 24 hr. urinary ketosteroid and hydroxycorticosteroid determination are indicated.

POTASSIUM....if high (above 5.0), be sure to rule out the more serious causes such as diabetes, metabolic acidosis, kidney disease, or lung disease. As mentioned, hypoadrenalism is associated with a high serum potassium. In most cases, this potassium elevation is not due to diet or supplements but is caused by a leakage of potassium from the cells into the bloodstream.

POTASSIUM....if low (below 3.7), think first of severe cellular potassium deficiency, since this can lead to fatal cardiac arrhythmia (especially if levels fall below 3.5). If the patient has diarrhea or is vomiting, this is the likely cause since much potassium can be lost through the digestive juices. Use raw honey, 1/3 cup three to four times daily. Many honeys, especially dark ones, are rich in potassium. Honey will stop diarrhea by holding water and digestive juices within the gut and helps the immune system eradicate the infection or eliminate the toxin.

Be sure to evaluate the patient's diet. Diets high in refined foods eventually cause a potassium deficiency. By the time blood levels become lowered, the cells have become extremely deficient. Ask about drug usage. Diuretic use is one of the most common causes of low potassium.

Treatment should consist of potassium supplements as either citrate, acetate, or aspartate. Avoid potassium chloride tablets (Slow-K, etc.) since their use is associated with a high incidence of gastric and/or intestinal ulcerations. Foods rich in potassium should be added liberally to the diet. These include:

almonds	papaya
apricots, dried	paprika
bananas, especially plantain	parsley
basil	parsnips
brazil nuts	peaches, dried
cabbage	peanuts
cantaloupe	pecans

cashews
chestnuts
dates
dill weed
hazelnuts
honey (darker varieties)
honeydew melon
mango
molasses (blackstrap)

pomegranate
prunes
raisins
red pepper
soybean flour
squash (the winter variety is
    particularly high)
tomatoes (especially tomato juice)
turmeric
watermelon

URIC ACID....if high (above 7.5), think impaired protein synthesis or utilization. Uric acid is a by-product of nucleic acid metabolism. Nucleic acids are the nuclear materials (i.e. RNA and DNA) used by the body to initiate the synthesis of proteins. A high uric acid level may indicate that proteins are being broken down too rapidly. Sugar increases uric acid levels, probably by causing tissue destruction or by increasing the rate at which proteins are broken down. High uric acid may also indicate the need for supplemental folic acid, since folates are involved in the metabolism of nucleic acids. A recent study showed that supplementation with folic acid decreased elevated levels.

Medical conditions associated with elevated uric acid levels include gout, kidney disease, diuretic overuse, diabetes, asthma, rheumatoid arthritis, hyperparathyroidism, and liver disease.

Treatment should include removal of all sources of refined sugar. Foods rich in potassium, magnesium, and folates should be prescribed. Vitamin C, E, A, and other antioxidants should be added. It is interesting to note that uric acid itself has antioxidant-like functions. A large glass of freshly squeezed vitamin A rich vegetable juice, such as carrot-parsley juice can also be taken daily.

URIC ACID....if low (below 4.0), think first of folic acid deficiency. A lack of uric acid means that not enough nuclear material is being synthesized. Folic acid, and to a lesser degree, B-12, are the key nutrients in this sequence. Adding 5 to 30 mgs. of folic acid daily often brings the uric acid to normal. If you see levels as low as 2.5, severe folic acid deficiency is likely. Add chlorella, the richest known source of RNA, 15 to 20 tablets three times daily. Other foods rich in RNA/DNA include:

sardines
chicken
liver

other cold water fish
turkey
wheat or rice germ

Many of the above foods are also rich in antioxidants. Beta carotene, selenium, and vitamin E protect RNA and DNA from damage by radiation and toxic compounds. Their intake should be increased when uric acid levels are abnormal.

BILIRUBIN (Total or Direct)....if either of these are elevated, evidence of severe liver disease exists. Viral hepatitis should be the first concern, although cancer and other obstructive liver diseases are possible.

Treatment is difficult in the case of obstructive diseases. If the diagnosis of viral hepatitis is confirmed, various foods and herbs which purge bile out of the liver may be utilized. The most valuable of these is the juice of beets. An 8 oz. glass of beet juice, combined with a quarter cup of olive oil and the juice of one whole lemon or lime (that is, if the patient is not citrus intolerant) could help lower bilirubin levels by increasing fecal bile content. Silymarin, as described in Chapter 8, helps seal off liver cell damage and prevents further damage from occurring. In addition, use large doses of antioxidants to help the body control the growth of the virus and to assist the immune system in destroying it. These antioxidants also act to prevent the breakdown of red cell membranes, which will further aggravate the bilirubin levels.

BILIRUBIN (Total)....if decreased (below .2), think first of anemia due to iron deficiency. Less bilirubin is being made because fewer red cells are available for turnover. Barbituates and aspirin derivatives may lower bilirubin measurements.

BILIRUBIN (Indirect)....if high (above .9), it is likely that more bilirubin is being formed than the body can get rid of. Several types of anemia including hereditary types increase indirect bilirubin. In these conditions, red blood cells are being rapidly destroyed due to their abnormal shape and function. Inflammatory conditions throughout the body, as well as hepatic inflammation, may also be responsible. If the indirect bilirubin is the only form elevated, it is likely that the patient has a malfunctioning, inflamed liver. Treatment would be the same as with elevated total bilirubin, with the addition of bioflavonoids, ginger root, turmeric, fish oils, and other anti-inflammatory nutrients.

TRIGLYCERIDES....if the fasting sample is high (above 150), think first of carbohydrate excess or alcoholism. I often recommend both fasting and post-prandial triglyceride measurements. It is a good idea to see how the body reacts to the norms of life. Levels above 250 indicate severe carbohydrate intolerance. Deficiencies of chromium, niacin, biotin, thiamine, inositol, and magnesium are likely. Essential fatty acid deficiency is another important factor. Hypothyroidism must always be ruled out since this leads to a defect in how rapidly sugars and starches are metabolized.

Reduce all dietary sources of carbohydrates and watch the triglycerides drop. Carnitine and niacin are most helpful in increasing the rate of fat clearance from the blood stream, and its resultant combustion into fuel by the cells. Add to the diet foods rich in carnitine including avocado, lamb, beef, and chicken. Rice bran would help since it is high in fiber and rich in thiamine and chromium. Chromium, if well absorbed, can cause a dramatic reduction in triglyceride levels.

In stubborn cases, check for food intolerance. Allergies to sugar, molasses, malt, etc. can cause elevated triglyceride levels.

TRIGLYCERIDES....if low (below 50), think of liver malfunction. A certain amount of fats in the blood are normal. Fats are needed as a source of fuel for organs such as the heart and kidneys. The liver makes proteins for carrying triglycerides to these organs. Abnormally low triglyceride levels often indicate poor protein synthesis in the liver or impaired hepatic synthesis of fatty acids. Such patients need high doses of essential fatty acids and also the B-vitamins used in protein and fatty acid synthesis. These include lecithin, linoleic acid, biotin, vitamin B-6, niacin, and pantothenic acid. A triglyceride level below 40 is a strong indication of essential fatty acid deficiency. Zinc is needed before essential fatty acids can be properly utilized. Up to 100 mgs. daily may be helpful. A word of caution — large doses of zinc should not be administered without monitoring the red blood count. In susceptible individuals, too much zinc can cause a copper-deficiency anemia. This occurs because excess zinc blocks the absorption of copper from the gut.

On the other hand, some liver diseases (e.g., Wilson's disease) are associated with extremely high blood and liver levels of copper. In this instance, high doses of zinc would be of exceptional value.

CHOLESTEROL.....if high (above 205), first check for excess dietary carbohydrate. If this is not the case, consider that there exists an increased need for antioxidant protection. Cholesterol is one of the most important antioxidants made by the body. It protects cell membranes from all sorts of noxious insults. An elevated cholesterol level despite a low carbohydrate diet indicates the existence of oxidative damage to cell membranes. As a rule, the higher the cholesterol, the greater the free radical activity. Try to find what is causing the elevated free radical activity. Increase dosages of all antioxidants, particularly vitamin E, beta carotene, and selenium, and watch the cholesterol drop.

Cholesterol is a critical component of cell membranes. It is needed for membrane synthesis and repair. Any process which damages cell membranes may cause a secondary rise in cholesterol levels.

Nutrients which help lower cholesterol levels include niacin, carnitine, vitamin C, taurine, lecithin, and fiber. Garlic, onion, chlorella, and shiitake mushroom extract all contain substances which help normalize cholesterol synthesis in the liver. Large doses of fish oils (greater than 3.0 grams daily) can be helpful, as is olive oil which lowers cholesterol levels better than polyunsaturates. But the most important of all is to change the diet and eliminate all sources of refined sugar and starch, including alcohol.

CHOLESTEROL....if decreased (below 160), this may be a sign of immune decline. Think also of adrenal insufficiency. Levels below 130 are highly correlated with cancer. Normalizing low cholesterol levels is often difficult. Squalene is a precursor to cholesterol synthesis. It is found in high amounts in the livers of sharks. Sharks almost never get cancer. There is no evidence as of yet that supplemental squalene raises depressed cholesterol levels. Pure, extra-virgin oil also contains squalene. Lowered cholesterol may be an indication of severe manganese deficiency. This could be revealed by a hair analysis, or a whole blood manganese level. As of yet, there is no first-class test available for assessing manganese nutrition. Regardless, foods rich in manganese should be added to the diet. These include:

almonds	avocados
beets	beet tops
blackberries	blueberries
boysenberries	Brazil nuts
chard, Swiss	chestnuts (fresh)
coconut	figs (dried)
ginger	green beans
lettuce	lima beans
liver	loganberries
navy beans	parsley
peaches, dried	peanuts
pears, dried	persimmons
pineapple	potatoes
raisins	raspberries
rice bran and polishings	soybeans
spices	spinach
strawberries	sunflower seeds
turnip greens	walnuts
wheat germ	whole grain flours

Absorption of manganese from wheat, rye and oats and other grains may be compromised due to the existence of phytates, which bind minerals so tightly that they cannot be easily absorbed. A similar problem may exist with nuts, which are the richest food source of manganese. Therefore, fruits, vegetables, and meats constitute the best sources, since the manganese they contain is more easily digested and assimilated.

Other nutrients important for the metabolism of cholesterol include thiamine, vitamin C, lipoic acid, and essential fatty acids. One of the early signs of essential fatty acid deficiency is an increased cholesterol level. Later, however, the cholesterol often falls well below the normal range. If cholesterol levels are persistently low, check for other signs of essential fatty acid deficiency such as dry skin, constipation, eczema, dry or oily hair, etc.

A significant ill-effect of lowered cholesterol is reduced adrenal hormone synthesis. Without cholesterol, the hormones of the adrenal cortex cannot be produced. The consequences may be disasterous. Without adrenal cortical hormones, diseases ranging from arthritis to fatal cardiac arrhythmia can develop. There is another serious side effect — immune decay. A complex interaction exists between adrenal hormones and immune function. It is well known that patients with Addison's disease, the extreme of adrenal failure, are vulnerable to all sorts of infections. If left untreated, such patients can die from infections by opportunistic microorganisms.

A very low cholesterol must not be taken lightly, and in some ways is more ominous than high levels. I advise anyone with a cholesterol level below 150 to 160 to eat foods rich in cholesterol, including liver, sweetbreads, eggs, beef, lamb, butter, whole milk, and cheese.

CALCIUM...if high (above 10.2), think first of mobilization of excess amounts of calcium from bone (*secondary hyperparathyroidism*). This can be caused by aluminum toxicity, lithium carbonate therapy, and vitamin D or even calcium deficiency. Often, a dose of 1500 to 2000 mgs. of absorbable calcium with vitamin D (the best source of vitamin D is cod liver oil) will bring the calcium to normal. Other trace minerals such as magnesium, zinc, copper, and manganese are needed to maintain bone density, as is vitamin A.

Refined sugar causes the mobilization of calcium and magnesium from bone. This can result in either high or low serum calcium values. Although much ado has been made concerning the possible connection of high protein diets with osteoporosis, refined sugar is the primary culprit in this respect. The consumption of refined sugar dramatically increases the mobilization of trace minerals from bone. Do not worry about reducing protein intake. Cut back on the carbohydrates first, and, if that doesn't work, modify protein consumption.

CALCIUM....if decreased (below 9.0), a calcium deficiency exists. However, this can be caused by a variety of factors, including:

1. low stomach acid output *(hypochlorhydria)*
2. vitamin D deficiency
3. dietary calcium deficiency
4. kidney disease
5. pregnancy (all the calcium is being used up)
6. hypoparathyroidism
7. maldigestion of protein

8. liver dysfunction

9. alcoholic gastritis

The liver makes proteins (e.g. albumin) which act to bind and carry calcium. If the patient does not respond to supplementation with calcium (1500 to 2000 mgs. per day) and vitamin D (two tablespoons of cod liver oil daily), the liver is probably defective in protein synthesis. This would be confirmed by borderline-low levels of serum albumin and/or globulin.

PHOSPHORUS....if high (above 4.2), think dietary excess (soft drinks are high in phosphates, as are red meats). Persistent elevations may indicate kidney dysfunction, and chronic infection in the kidneys is possible. In addition, both the parathyroid glands and liver manage phosphorus nutrition. Hypofunction of the parathyroids is possible.

PHOSPHORUS....if decreased (below 2.5), think vitamin D deficiency. Reduced secretion of gastric juices, especially hydrochloric acid is possible. Low phosphorus is also seen in diabetes and liver disease. Be sure the diet is rich in high-phosphorus foods which include fish, red meats, poultry, eggs, cheese, nuts, seeds, rice bran, soybeans, and peanut butter. In addition, supplement the diet with two tablespoons of cod-liver oil daily for at least one month. Increased exposure to sunlight, especially for the elderly, may be necessary.

ALKALINE PHOSPHATASE....if elevated (above 110), think first of liver disease. A heavy concentration of this enzyme is found in the liver, although it is prevalent in bone and intestinal mucosa. Disease or destruction of any of these tissues leads to elevated levels. Your first thought should be either obstructive liver disease or bone disease. Cancer metastases to the bone should be ruled out. However, a wide range of conditions can lead to elevated alkaline phosphatase levels. Be sure also to check the patient's medication list, since drug-induced liver toxicity is a most likely cause. The level in children is normally elevated due to bone growth.

ALKALINE PHOSPHATASE....if low (below 45), think of zinc deficiency. Zinc is a cofactor for this enzyme, and enzyme synthesis is dependent upon adequate tissue levels of it. Folic acid deficiency may also lead to reduced levels. It is likely that protein digestion in general is impaired. Give 50 to 100 mgs. of zinc and 5 or more mgs. of folic acid daily.

LIVER ENZYMES (SGOT, SGPT)....if high (above 40), think of inflammation of the liver (i.e. hepatitis). This condition is usually caused by an infection, although toxic chemicals can cause a form of hepatitis.

Remember that one of the primary functions of the liver is to detoxify various chemicals and poisons. Whenever there is an exposure to noxious chemicals, they are concentrated specifically in the liver.

In either case, large doses of antioxidants are needed. Beet juice or powder may help heal the liver and decrease enzyme levels. There are many natural substances which have been discovered to heal liver damage and lower elevated enzyme levels. A few of them are mentioned below:

- raw or crude liver extract
- lipoic acid
- thiamine (as Allithiamine)
- lecithin
- choline
- methionine

- garlic extract
- chlorella
- biotin
- vitamin E
- cysteine
- selenium

In addition, many herbs have a protective effect upon liver cells. Silymarin, turmeric, licorice root, ginger, and ginseng are a few examples. Elevations of SGOT have been associated with selenium deficiency, and increasing tissue stores of this mineral offers significant protection. It is likely that this effect is due to increased synthesis of glutathione peroxidase by hepatocytes.

It is important to note that 30% or more of the weight of the liver is made up of *Kupffer* cells. These are phagocytic cells which clear debris, toxins and microorganisms *before* they can do damage. When these cells begin to malfunction, they can become easily overwhelmed and all sorts of health problems can result. Their proper function is dependent upon an adequate supply of a variety of nutrients. Vitamins A, C, E, B-vitamins, selenium, zinc and essential fatty acids are especially important. If liver enzymes are elevated, Kupffer cells are being overloaded and viral, bacterial, fungal, and even parasitic infection can run rampant throughout the body and/or within the liver itself. In addition, carbohydrate intolerance may lead to elevated liver enzymes. This is a result of the liver being infiltrated by fat. This fatty infiltration results when excess dietary carbohydrates are synthesized into triglycerides and other storage forms of fat. Do not take mild elevations of liver enzymes lightly.

GLOBULIN....if high (above 3.3), think first of hypertrophy of the lymphoid tissue within the bone marrow or lymphatic system. On a more serious scale, this could represent the existence of lymphoid tumors. The liver is also involved in globulin synthesis. Therefore, inflammatory diseases of the liver, especially mononucleosis and hepatitis, should be ruled out. Persistent elevations in globulin levels lead to the suspicion of viral replication within B-lymphocytes, which causes dysfunctional antibody synthesis. Infections by parasites or bacteria are also possible. Large doses of nutrients which nourish the immune system and liver may be needed. Vitamin A (2 to 3 tablespoons of cod-liver oil daily) could quiet down the B-lymphocyte proliferation. Selenium, zinc, calcium, magnesium, and manganese are also important, as are the B-vitamins, especially B-5, B-6, and folic acid.

GLOBULIN....if low (below 2.3), think of impaired globulin synthesis by the liver and B-lymphocytes. Most people with low globulin levels are deficient in manganese and other minerals. These minerals cannot be properly absorbed or transported in the blood without globulin proteins. It is likely that the immune system is under pressure and a chronic viral or yeast infection is almost assured. When globulin levels drop below 2.0, the body becomes vulnerable to invasion by opportunistic micro-organisms. This includes colonization of the mucous membranes by Candida Albicans or various parasites, such as Giardia or ameobas. The liver also becomes much more susceptible to becoming infected.

Raising the globulin level often poses a challenge. Liberating the immune system from chronic infections is the prime objective. This, of course, takes time. Improving the function of the thyroid and adrenal glands will help. Low globulin may also be a signal of systemic vitamin A deficiency. Look for other signs, such as dry or scaly skin, follicular hyperkeratosis (skin that looks like "gooseflesh"), vision disturbances, night blindness, brittle hair, pitted or decayed teeth, chronic diarrhea, etc. Give cod liver oil, 1 tablespoon twice daily, reducing this dosage to a tablespoon every other day once the deficiency is corrected. In addition, some studies have shown that high doses of folic acid and vitamin B-5 (pantothenic acid) raise globulin levels. The likely mechanism is increased globulin synthesis by B-lymphocytes. In this respect, it would be wise to add vitamin B-12, since it is also required for globulin synthesis to proceed.

If a cardiac patient has a low globulin level beware — their ability to transport minerals may be impaired. In such a patient, I suggest the dose of heart-healing minerals such as calcium, magnesium, copper, zinc and manganese be doubled. These minerals are far more valuable in maintaining the health of the heart than any drug or surgical procedure.

HDL CHOLESTEROL....if low (below 40), think first of liver dysfunc-tion. The liver synthesizes most of the HDL fraction found in the body. Improved liver function will automatically result in an increase in the liver's ability to synthesize proteins such as HDL. In addition, the following is a list of nutrients which have been proven to increase HDL levels:

- chromium
- garlic extract
- carnitine
- fish oils

- flax seed oil
- niacin
- vitamin C

- lecithin
- olive oil
- vitamin E

3. ACCURATE TESTS TO HELP CONFIRM THE DIAGNOSIS

SUSPICION	IDEAL TEST	LAB
Food allergies	Food Intolerance	N.T.L.
Vitamin B-1 deficiency	Red Cell Transketolase	N.T.L.
Vitamin B-2 dysfunction	Red Cell Glutathione Reductase	N.T.L.
Vitamin B-3 deficiency	Urinary NAD	(not yet available)
Vitamin B-6 dysfunction	Red Cell Glutamate Pyruvate Transaminase	N.T.L.
Manganese deficiency	Isocitrate Dehydrogenase	(not yet available)
Magnesium deficiency	Red Cell Magnesium Level	Reference labs
Iron deficiency	Serum Iron and Ferritin	Reference labs
Selenium deficiency	Red Cell Glutathione Peroxidase	N.T.L.
Impaired antioxidant function	Red Cell Glutathione Peroxidase & Reductase	N.T.L.
Glutathione deficiency	Red Cell Glutathione Peroxidase	N.T.L.

Highly accurate tests for cellular deficiency of vitamins A, C, E, B-3, B-5, folic acid, vitamin B-12, and biotin are yet to be developed. Serum vitamin A, folic acid, and B-12 values are useful in the case of extreme deficiency only. Hair analysis may reveal trends of mineral absorption. Clinically valuable blood tests for zinc, manganese, chromium, and other trace minerals are lacking.

Note: The address for N.T.L. (Nutritional Testing Laboratories) is 1401 W. Golf Rd., Suite 404, Rolling Meadows, IL. 60008. Ph. (708) 640-1377. Reference Labs such as Damon, Med-Path, and Smith-Kline are available in any major city in the U.S.A.

APPENDIX A

Nutritional Content of
Selected Foods

While reviewing these charts, keep in mind one important fact —there is no way to standardize the nutritional content of any given food. The nutritional value of foods vary with growing conditions, soil nutrient content, and freshness. The most critical factor is the nutrient content of the soil in which the food is grown. These charts are approximations to the best of human ability. For example, a carrot grown in California will have a selenium or vitamin A content different from one grown in Wisconsin — illustrating that there is no "standardized carrot."

CHART #1

There has been a great deal of discussion in the last few years concerning the health benefits of bran. This chart illustrates the nutritional value of two of the most popular sources of bran. Wheat germ is listed instead of wheat bran, since its nutritional value is considerably greater. Bran also contains trace minerals such as selenium, silicon, chromium, and manganese, but levels have yet to be accurately determined.

254

% of U.S. RDA per equivalent weight	RICE BRAN	WHEAT GERM	OAT BRAN
Thiamine	60	20	20
Riboflavin	6	8	6
Niacin	50	6	1
Vitamin B-6	8	10	Not detectable
Vitamin E	15	8	Not detectable
Iron	15	10	10
Phosphorus	45	25	20
Magnesium	60	15	15
Zinc	10	20	8

As you can see from the above, rice bran is a far better source of most nutrients than either wheat germ or oat bran. In addition, rice bran contains a special oil which apparently helps lower cholesterol levels. Both rice and oat bran are rich sources of fiber and can be used as a fiber supplement.

CHART #2
FOODS HIGH IN MAGNESIUM

I have listed food sources of magnesium since the majority of the population is deficient in it. The likelihood that deficiency exists is increased in those who have symptoms such as muscle spasms or twitches, rapid heartbeat, or arrhythmia, poor appetite, nausea, and confusion.

There are many food sources of magnesium. The following chart lists magnesium in foods as milligrams per equivalent weight.

Rice bran 785
Coriander leaf, dried 694
Dillweed, dried 451
Celery seed 440
Sage 428
Mustard, dried 422

Basil 422
Cocoa powder 420
Fennel seed 385
Wheat germ, toasted 364
Tarragon 347
Brazil nuts 318
Soybean flour, defatted 318
Almonds 293
Molasses, blackstrap 258
Spinach, frozen 104
Chickpeas, dry or canned 54
Apricots, dried 50

Other excellent food sources include black eyed peas, cashews, pecans, bananas, beet greens, avocados, filberts, tofu, oatmeal, and buckwheat. Foods which are organically grown contain up to 10 times more magnesium than foods that are grown commercially. Using lots of spices is one of the easiest ways to get extra magnesium. A good rule of thumb is this; the hotter the spice, the more magnesium it contains.

CHART #3
SELENIUM CONTENT OF FOODS

The selenium content of foods varies from region to region. This variation is entirely dependent upon the amount of selenium within the soil. The chart below illustrates just how wide of a variation this can be. The figures marked with an @ are foods which were grown in Maryland, a region with relatively low amounts of selenium. Those marked with an * describe foods grown in South Dakota, a high-selenium area. Figures marked with a + describe foods from Venezuela, another region with selenium-rich soils. All foods were analyzed for selenium content by the U.S. Department of Agriculture.

FOOD	AMOUNT	SELENIUM RANGES (in micrograms)
Carrots, raw	1	1.8@ to 105 *
Cabbage, shredded	1/2 cup	1.8@ to 316 *
Onion, raw	1/2 cup	1.3@ to 1513 *
Potatoes, raw	1 large	1.0@ to 235 *
Tomatoes, raw	1	0.7@ to 165 *
Cheese	1.5 oz.	3.8@ to 18 +
Egg	1 large	5.0@ to 87 +
Chicken breast	4 oz.	13.0@ to 79 +

From the above chart, it becomes clear that *all food is not the same.*

While a head of cabbage from South Dakota and Maryland look alike, their nutrient content is vastly different. If you have lived on the East or Northwestern coast of the United States, or in the Great Lakes region for much of your life, you have been getting only a minute amount of selenium from food grown there — *barely enough to keep you alive!* Such individuals should make it a point to include selenium-rich foods in the diet on a daily basis. A selection of selenium-rich food includes garlic, organ meats, butter, fish, lobster, crab, clams, lamb, nuts, wheat germ, fresh whole wheat flour, cider vinegar, mushrooms, Swiss chard, radishes, turnips, and mushrooms.

CHART #4
HIGHEST FOOD SOURCES OF VITAMIN E

Only a few foods contain appreciable amounts of vitamin E. Vitamin E is found in the highest concentration within foods which are naturally rich in oils. In addition, certain vegetables, such as spinach, tomatoes, and sweet potatoes contain valuable amounts.

FOOD	PORTION	VITAMIN E (I.U.)
Wheat germ oil	1 tbsp.	37.2
Sunflower seeds	1/4 cup	26.8
Wheat germ, raw	1/2 cup	12.8
Sunflower seed oil	1 tbsp.	12.7
Almonds	1/4 cup	12.7
Pecans	1/4 cup	12.7
Hazelnuts	1/4 cup	12.5
Safflower oil	1 tbsp.	7.9
Peanuts	1/4 cup	4.9
Sweet Potato	1 small	4.8
Spinach, cooked	1 cup	4.5
Lobster	3 oz.	2.3
Salmon steak	3 oz.	2.0

The above chart illustrates the difficulty of trying to get adequate amounts of vitamin E through the diet alone. Unless you consume two or more tablespoons of wheat germ oil daily or are eating sunflower seeds by the handful, you need supplemental vitamin E. The minimum recommended dose for most people is 400 I.U. daily.

CHART #5
FOOD SOURCES OF BIOTIN

Rich Sources
- kidney
- liver
- soybean flour

Good Sources
- cauliflower
- cocoa bean
- eggs
- mushrooms
- peanuts
- peanut butter
- almonds
- beef
- veal
- halibut
- mackerel
- sardines
- lobster

Fair Sources
- chicken
- carrots
- spinach
- most fruits
- collards
- kale
- spinach
- Swiss chard
- watercress
- kiwi fruit

CHART #6
FOOD SOURCES OF FOLIC ACID

Rich Sources
- liver and other
  organ meats
- wheat bran
- rice bran
- rice germ

Good Sources
- nuts
- soybean flour
- mushrooms
- oranges
- cantaloupe
- strawberries
- salmon
- blue cheese
- eggs
- wild rice
- brown rice
- buckwheat flour
- lobster
- sunflower seeds

Fair Sources
- chicken
- broccoli
- sweet red peppers
- whole wheat flour
- avocados

The folic acid found in eggs and meat is absorbed better than that found in grains, vegetables, and nuts. This should be kept in mind when making food choices based on this chart. Folic acid is easily destroyed by cooking, particularly by boiling. Anywhere between 40 to 95% of the original amount of folic acid found in fruits and/or vegetables is lost during canning and cooking primarily because much of the water is discarded, and folic acid is water soluble. However, if the cooking water is retained as in soup or sauces, or is drunk, much of the folic acid will be recovered.

CHART #7
FOOD SOURCES OF PYRIDOXINE (Vitamin B-6)

Rich Sources	Good Sources	Fair Sources
• rice bran	• avocados	• eggs
• wheat bran	• bananas	• milk
• sunflower seeds	• corn	• mangos
	• fish	• cantaloupe
	• kidney	• pineapple
	• liver	• figs, dried
	• lean meat	
	• nuts	
	• wild rice	
	• brown rice	
	• soy beans	
	• whole grain flour	

CHART #8
FOOD SOURCES OF VITAMIN B-12

Vitamin B-12 is the largest and most complex of all known vitamins. There are few dietary sources of this important vitamin even though little, if any, is made within the body. Meats and dairy products constitute the majority of dietary intake. This is because vitamin B-12 originates from bacteria which live in the intestines of animals. These bacteria are found in large amounts primarily in the first stomach (the lumen) of herbivorous animals such as cows, goats, and sheep. Bacteria synthesize this structurally complex vitamin within the lumen, from which it is absorbed into the bloodstream to be taken to various organs and tissues. This is why organ meats, muscle meats, eggs, and milk products constitute significant dietary sources. Fish and seafood consume B-12 through a secondary source—dark green algae, such as chlorella, the richest known plant source of B-12.

Richest Natural Sources	Excellent Sources	Good Sources
• lamb liver	• roe (fish eggs) from cod, haddock or herring	• catfish
• beef liver	• mackerel	• tuna
• lamb kidney	• cod	• halibut
• beef kidney	• crab	• lamb
• turkey liver	• eggs	• beef
	• sardines	• cheese
	• mozzarella cheese	
	• herring	
	• salmon	
	• chlorella	

CHART #9
FOOD SOURCES OF VITAMIN C

Richest Natural Sources	Excellent Sources	Good Sources
• acerola cherry and rose hips	• guavas	• broccoli
	• strawberries	• limes
	• oranges	• black currants
	• grapefruit	• green peppers
	• lemons	• red peppers
		• parsley
		• turnip greens
		• mustard greens
		• avocados
		• melons
		• papaya
		• Brussels sprouts
		• red cabbage
		• cauliflower
		• collards
		• kale
		• spinach
		• Swiss chard
		• watercress
		• kiwi fruit

CHART #10
SUGAR CONTENT OF FRUITS

Fruit contains the natural sugars fructose and glucose with fructose usually being found in the highest concentration. These sugars are bound to cellulose and other fibers within the whole fruit. This allows the sugars to be released gradually into the bloodstream from which they are delivered to the cells to be used as a source of fuel. The following chart lists the percentages of natural sugar found in fruits:

5-7% NATURAL SUGAR
- cantaloupe
- honeydew
- papaya
- strawberries
- watermelon

8-9% NATURAL SUGAR
- grapefruit
- lemon
- lime

10-12% NATURAL SUGAR
- apricots
- blackberries
- currants
- oranges
- peaches
- tangerines

15-16% NATURAL SUGAR
- apples
- blueberries
- cherries
- grapes
- kumquats
- loganberries
- pears
- pineapple
- raspberries

20% OR MORE NATURAL SUGAR
- apple juice
- bananas
- dates
- figs
- raisins
- grape juice
- orange juice

1. ORDERING INFORMATION FOR NUTRITIONAL FOODS AND SUPPLEMENTS

NUTRITIONAL PRODUCTS   **ORDERING INFORMATION**

Additives-Free Frozen Dinners
(Taste Great Too!)

OVEN POPPERS
405 Spruce Street
Manchester, NH 03103
Call Collect 603-644-3773
603-644-3773
Call Collect

Allithiamine
B-Complex

CARDIOVASCULAR RESEARCH
1061-B Shary Circle
Concord, California 94518
(415) 827-2636

Herbal Garlic,
Digestive Enzymes

Ms. Georgia Janish
5300 Hwy. 14W
Janesville, Wisconsin
(608) 756-2244

Basic H
Pro-Lecin Nibblers

PHYSICIAN'S HEALTH DESIGN
804 Loretta Dr.
Goodlettsville, Tennessee 37072
(615) 859-7846

Balancing Infusion,
Shampure

NUTRITIONAL SUPPLEMENT
SERVICE
212 Willow Parkway
Buffalo Grove, Illinois 60089
(800) 243-5242

Bromelain
Biotin

GY&N PRODUCTS
c/o Nutritional Supplement
Service
(800) 243-5242

Chlorella (Sun Chlorella)
and Wakasa

YSK International
(Available at
many health-food stores)
or by mail order
1-800-243-5242

Chromium Picolinate Coat's Aloe (Pur Aloe), Aloe Gel	NUTRITIONAL SUPPLEMENT SERVICE (800) 243-5242
Deodorized Garlic Extract	NUTRITIONAL SUPPLEMENT SERVICE 212 Willow Parkway Buffalo Grove, Illinois 60089 (800) 243-5242
Lipoic acid (ask for "Thioctic")	CARDIOVASCULAR RESEARCH (415) 827-2636
Fish Oils (EPA/DHA) ask for "Kyolic-EPA"	KYOLIC-WAKUNAGA CORP. Mission Viejo, California (800) 421-2998
Premium-Grade Vitamin E	NUTRITIONAL SUPPLEMENT SERVICE (800) 243-5242
Premium-Grade Beta Carotene	NUTRITIONAL SUPPLEMENT SERVICE (800) 243-5242
Selenium (Yeast Free) ask for Sea-SEL-Kelp or Selenomethionine	SCIENTIFIC CONSULTING SERVICES (800) 333-7414 KLAIRE LABS (800) 533-7255, ext. 100
Supercholine	CARDIOVASCULAR RESEARCH (415) 827-2636
Tanalbit, Taurine or Tyrosine	SCIENTIFIC CONSULTING SERVICES (800) 333-7414
Medi-Plex Hair Loss Regimen	MEDI-PLEX 2730 Wilshire Blvd., Suite 301 Santa Monica, California 90403 (800) 292-6006

FOOD PRODUCTS	ORDERING INFORMATION

FOOD PRODUCTS

DR. BRONNER'S
SEASONING, BOUILLON
& VINEGAR

Box 28
Escondido, California 92025

(found in many health-food stores)

KEFIR

LIFEWAY FOODS
Skokie, Illinois

(may be found in grocery and/or health-food stores)

GROUND FLAX SEED

FORTIFIED FLAX
Omega-Life, Inc.
P.O. Box 208
Brookfield, Wisconsin 53008-0208

FLAX SEED OIL

ALLERGY RESOURCES, INC.
175 Huntington Beach Drive
Colorado Springs, Colorado 80921
(800) USE-FLAX

HAZELNUT BUTTER &
HAZELNUTS, ROASTED
— ALL NATURAL

HENRY'S FARMS
1216 E. Henry Road
Newberg, Oregon 97132
(503) 538-5244

NATURAL-ORGANIC
BUFFALO MEAT

U.S. BISON COMPANY
W11282 Wildlife Road
Withee, Wisconsin 54498
(800) 225-7457

WATERFIER
Water Treatment Unit
&
SHOWER YOKE
Water Purifier for the Shower

O'MARA PRECISION BUILDERS
3130 Eugene Street
Burton, Michigan 48519
(313) 743-8650

WATER-PURIFYING STRAW

NUTRITIONAL SUPPLEMENT
SERVICE
(800) 243-5242

APPENDIX C

CASSETTE TAPES

THE "EAT RIGHT" SERIES

1. How to Eat Right #1: At Home and the Grocery Store

2. How to Eat Right #2: While Travelling and Dining

3. Disease Prevention I: The Major Killers — Heart Disease, Cancer, Diabetes, Stroke and Alcoholism

4. Disease Pevention II: The Other Killers — Arthritis, Obesity, Lupus, Alzheimer's Hypothyroidism, Infection, and Adrenal Disorders

5. Preventing Aging: Diet, Supplements, and Other Nutritional Pearls

This series is available for $39.95 plus sales tax. Please add $2.50 shipping and handling.
Individual tapes are $9.95 plus $2.00 shipping and handling.
Payable by check or money order only.
Make payable to: A.I.C.M. c/o Cedar Graphics
1500-20th Street S.W.
Cedar Rapids, Iowa 52404

Note: No Tapes can be shipped to P.O. Boxes

ORDER FORM

ITEM	QTY.	AMOUNT
a. tape no. 1	_____	$ _____
b. tape no. 2	_____	$ _____
c. tape no. 3	_____	$ _____
d. tape no. 4	_____	$ _____
e. tape no. 5	_____	$ _____
f. tape series	_____	$ _____
g. book "Eat Right or Die Young"	_____	$ _____
Sub-Total		$ _____
Sales Tax (if any)		$ _____
Total		$ _____

ORDER BY C.O.D., VISA, MASTERCARD, OR CHECK
(C.O.D. charges are $3.35 additional). MAKE PAYABLE TO:

A.I.C.M. c/o Cedar Graphics
1500-20th Street S.W.
Cedar Rapids, Iowa 52404
Phone (319) 366-5335

For Visa/Mastercard, use the following form:

Card #_____ Exp. Date_____

Signature_____

Name _____

Address_____

City_____ State _____ Zip _____

BIBLIOGRAPHY

1. Aaseth, J., et al. 1980. Decreased levels of selenium in alcoholic cirrhosis. *N.E.J.M.* Oct 16.

2. Abdullah, T.H., Kandil, O., ElKadi, A., et al. 1988. Garlic revisited: therapeutic for the major diseases of our times? *Nat'l Med. Assoc.* 80(4):439-45.

3. Ackerman, I.A., Weinstein, I.B., Kaplan, H.S. 1978. Cancer of the esophagus. In: *Cancer in China* (eds. H.S. Kaplan and A. Tsuchitani). New York: A.R. Liss, pp. 111-36.

4. Adetumbi, M.A., Lau, B.H.S. 1983. Allium Sativum (garlic) — a natural antibiotic. *Medical Hypotheses* 12:227-37.

5. Agharanya, J.C., Alonso, R., Wurtman, R.J. 1981. Changes in catecholamine excretion after short-term tyrosine ingestion in normally fed human subjects. *Am. J. Clin. Nutr.* 34:82-87.

6. Agharanya, J.C., Wurtman, R.J. 1982. Effect of acute administration of large neutral amino acids on urinary excretion of catecholamines. *Life Sciences* 30(9):739-46.

7. Airola, P. 1978. *The Miracle of Garlic.* Health Plus Publishers, Phoenix.

8. Alexander, M., et al. 1985. Oral beta carotene can increase the numbers of OKT4+ cells in human blood. *Immunology Letters* 9:221.

9. Ambrosio, G., Weisfeldt, M.L., Jacobus, W.E. 1987. Evidence for a reversible oxygen radical-mediated component of reperfusion injury: reduction by recombinent human superoxide dismutase administered at the time of reflow. *Circulation* 75(1): 282-91.

10. Amella, M., Bonner, C., Briancon, F., et al. 1985. Inhibition of mast cell histamine release by flavonoids and bioflavonoids. *Planta Medica* 51:16-20.

11. Ames, B. 1983. Dietary carcinogens and anti-carcinogens. *Science* 221:1256-64.

12. *Anonymous. 1987. Second opinions reduce by-pass surgery. Am. Med. News Oct. 2, p. 72.*

13. Augustine, G.J., Jr., Levitan, H. 1980. Neurotransmitter release from a vertebrate neuromuscular synapse affected by a food dye. *Science* 207: 1489-90.

14. Azuma, J., et al. 1985. Therapeutic effect of taurine in congestive heart failure: a double-blind crossover trail. *Clin. Cardiol.* 8:276:82.

15. Balentine, J.D. 1982. *Pathology of Oxygen Toxicity.* Academic Press, New York.

16. Beck, W.S. 1988. Cobalamin and the nervous system. *N.E.J.M.* 318:1752-54.

17. Becker, C.E., et al. 1976. Diagnosis and treatment of amanital phalloides-type mushroom poisoning: use of thioctic acid. *West. J. Med.* 125:100-09.

18. Beisel, W.R., Edelman, R., Nauss, K., Suskind, R. 1981. Single nutrient effects on immunologic function. *J.A.M.A.* 245:53.

19. Belizan, J.M., et al. 1983. Reduction of blood pressure with calcium supplementation in young adults. *J.A.M.A.* 249:1161-5.

20. Belman, S. 1983. Onion and garlic oil inhibit tumor growth. *Carcinogenesis* 4(8):1063-65.

21. Belsheim, J.A., Gnarpe, G.H. 1981. Antibiotics and granulocytes. Direct and indirect effects on granulocyte chemotaxis. *Acta. Path. Micro. Scand.* 89:217-21.

22. Benda, L., Dittrich, H., Ferenzi, P., et al. 1980. The influence of therapy with silymarin on the survival rate of patients with liver cirrhosis. *Wiener Klinishce Wochenschrift* Oct. 10, p. 678.

23. Berkow, S., Palmer, S. 1986. Nutrition in medical education: current status and future directions. *Amer. Inst. Nutr.* (study completed by the National Research Council for Food and Nutrition—National Academy of Sciences, 2101 Constitution Avenue N.W. Washington, D.C. 20418).

24. Bertram, J., Peng, A., Rundhaug, J. 1988. Carotenoids have intrinsic cancer chemopreventive action in 10T1 cells. *F.A.S.E.B.J.* 2:1413

25. Beutler, E., et al. 1985. Plasma glutathione in health and in patients with malignant disease. *J. Lab. Clin. Med.* 105:581-84.

26. Bever, B.O., Zahnd, G.R. 1979. Plants with oral hypoglycemic action. *Quar. J. Crude Drug Res.* 17:139-96.

27. Bishop, J.E. 1977. Deaths of 2 liquid protein dieters tied to unusual heart rhythm abnormalities. *The Wall Street Journal* Dec. 1, p. 8.

28. Bjarnason, I., et al. 1987. Blood and protein loss via small intestinal inflammation induced by non-steroidal anti-inflammatory drugs. *Lancet* 2:711.

29. Bjerve, K.S., Thoresen, L., Borsting, S. 1988. Linseed and cod liver oil induce rapid growth in a 7-year old girl with n-3 fatty acid deficiency. *J. Parent. Ent. Nutr.* 12:521-25.

30. Bland, J. 1978. *The Use of the Clinical Laboratory in Preventive Medicine.* Bellevue Redmond Medical Labs Inc., Tacoma, Wash.

31. Bland, J. 1982. *The Accessory Food Factors in Health Promotion.* Vol. 2. Keats Publishing Inc., New Canaan, Conn., pp. 1-25.

32. Bland, J. 1985. *Nutraerobics.* Harper & Row, San Francisco.

33. Bland, J. (ed.). 1985. *Yearbook of Nutritional Medicine.* Keats Publishing, Inc., New Canaan, Conn.

34. Blau, L.W. 1950. Cherry diet control for gout and arthritis. *Tex. Rep. Bio. Med.* 8:309-11.

35. Bliznakov, E.G. 1986. *The Miracle Nutrient—Coenzyme Q-10.* Bantam Books.

36. Bloom, W.L., Flinchum, D. 1960. Osteomalacia with pseudofractures caused by the ingestion of aluminum hydroxide. *J.A.M.A.* 174:1327.

37. Blume, E. 1986. Aflatoxin. *Nutrition Action Healthletter.* Vol. 13(8). Center for Science in the Public Interest, Washington, D.C.

38. Bombardelli, E., Cirstoni, A., Carruthers, M. 1982. The effect of acute and chronic (Panax) ginseng saponins treatment on adrenal function; biochemical and pharmacological. *Proceedings of 3rd International Ginseng Symposium* pp. 9-16.

39. Bonjour, J.B. 1977. Biotin in man's nutrition and therapy: a review. *Int. J. Vit. Nutr. Res.* 47:107-18.

40. Bordia, A., Bansal, H.C., Arora, S.K., et al. 1975. Effect of the essential oils of garlic and onion on alimentary hyperlipidemia. *Atherosclerosis* 21:15.

41. Bordia, A. 1981. Effect of garlic on blood lipids in patients with coronary heart disease. *Am. J. Clin. Nutr.* 34:2100.

42. Breneman, J.C. 1978. *Basics of Food Allergy*. Charles C. Thomas, Springfield, Ill.

43. Brittelli, M., Culik, R., Dashiell, O., et al. 1979. Skin absorption of hexafluoroacetone: teratogenic and lethal effects in the rat fetus. *Tox. Appl. Pharm.* 47:35-39.

44. Brock, K., Berry, G., Mock, P., et al. 1988. Nutrients in diet and plasma and risk of in situ cervical cancer. *J. Nat. Canc. Inst.* 80:580-85.

45. Bruce, W.R., Dion, P.W. 1981. Studies relating to a fecal mutagen. *Am. J. Clin. Nutr.* 35:2511-12.

46. Buist, R. 1984. *Food Intolerance: What It is and How to Cope With It.* Harper & Row, Sydney, Australia.

47. Burke, W.B. Jr. 1982. *Inositol: Nature's Anxiety Fighter*. Hawkes Publishing, Inc., Salt Lake City, Utah.

48. Burr, M., et al. 1987. Atrophic gastritis and vitamin C status in two towns with different stomach cancer death rates. *Br. J. Canc.* 56:163-67.

49. Burto, G.W., Foster, D.O., Perly, B., et al. 1985. Biological antioxidants. *Philos. Trans. R. Soc.* B. London (ed.) 311:565-78.

50. Burton, J. 1989. Dietary fatty acids and inflammatory skin disease. *Lancet* 1:27-31.

51. Busse, W.W., Kopp, D.E., Middleton, E. 1984. Flavonoid modulation of human neutrophil function. *J. Allergy Clin. Immunol.* 73:801-9.

52. Calabarese, E.J. 1981. *Nutritional and Environmental Toxicity: the Influence of Nutritional Status on Pollutant Toxicity and Carcinogenicity.* Vol. 1-2. John Wiley & Sons, Chichester.

53. Caporaso, N., Smith, S.M., Eng, R.H.K. 1983. Anti-fungal activity
     in human serum after ingestion of garlic allium-sativum.
     Antimicrob. Agents Chemother. 23(5):700-02.

54. Carrol, J.E. Brooke, M.H., Shumate, J.B. 1981. Carnitine intake
     and excretion in neuromuscular diseases. *Am. J. Clin. Nutr.*
     34:2693-8.

55. Chanarin, I., Stephenson, E. 1988. Vegetarian diet and cobalamin
     deficiency: their association with tuberculosis. *J. Clin. Path.*
     41:759-62.

56. Chen, L. 1988. Effects of diuretics on riboflavin status and urinary
     excretion. *F.A.S.E.B.J.* 2:1573.

57. Cheney, G. 1949. Rapid healing of peptic ulcers in patients
     receiving fresh cabbage juice. *California Medicine* 70(1):10-14.

58. Cheney, G. 1950. The nature of the antipeptic-ulcer factor.
     Stanford Med. Bull. 8(3):145-59.

59. Chow, C.K. 1979. Nutritional influence on cellular antioxidant
     defense systems. *Am. J. Clin. Nutr.* 32:1066-81.

60. Clark, D. 1957. The endocrine approach to the treatment of
     allergy. *Ann. West. Med. Surg.* 2(9):404-07.

61. Clark, A.J., Mossholder, M.S., Gates, R. 1987. Folacin status in
     adolescent females. *Am. J. Clin. Nutr.* 46:302-6.

62. Clausen, J. 1988. Chromium induced clinical improvement in
     symptomatic hypoglycemia. *Bio. Tr. Elem. Res.* 17:229-36.

63. Cleave, T.L., Campbell, G.D. 1969. *Diabetes, Coronary
     Thrombosis and the Saccharine Disease.* John Wright & Sons,
     Bristol, England.

64. Cloarec, M.J., et al. 1987. Alpha tocopherol: effect on plasma
     lipoproteins in hypercholesterolemic patients. *Isr. J. Med. Sci.*
     23(8):869-72.

65. Cody, V., Middleton, E., Harborne, J.B. (eds.) 1986. *Plant
     Flavonoids in Biology and Medicine—Biochemical,
     Pharmacological, and Structure-activity Relationships.* A.R. Liss,
     New York.

66. Coggeshall, J.C., Heggers, J.P., Robson, M.C., et al. 1985. Biotin status and plasma glucose in diabetics. *Annal. N.Y. Acad. Sci.* 447:38992.

67. Collins, E.B., Ardt, P. 1980. Inhibition of C. Albicans by lactobacilli and lactobacillic fermented dairy products. *F.E.M.S. Micro. Rev.* (Sept.), 46:343-56.

68. Cook, J.D., et al. 1974. Serum ferritin as a measure of iron in normal subjects. *Amer. J. Clin. Nutr.* 27:9681-87.

69. Coombs, R.R.A., Oldham, G. 1981. Early rheumatoid-like joint lesions in rabbits drinking cow's milk. *Int. Arch. Allergy Appl. Immunol.* 64:287.

70. Cornell, R., Walker, W.A. Isselbacher, K.J. 1971. Intestinal absorption of horseradish peroxidase. A cytochemical study. *Lab. Invest.* 25:42-8.

71. Cousins, N. 1986. Panic—the ultimate disease. *Holistic Medicine.* March/April.

72. Cox, R.A., Hoppel, C.I. 1973. Biosynthesis of carnitine and 4-N-trimethylaminobutyrate from lysine. *Biochem. J.* 136:1075-82.

73. Crittenden, P.J. 1948. Studies on the pharmacology of biotin. *Arch. Int. Pharmacodyn. Ther.* 76:263-75.

74. Cruikshank, J.M., Thorp, T.M., Zacharias, J.F. 1987. Benefits and potential harm of lowering high blood pressure. *Lancet* 1:581-83.

75. Curtis, A.C., Baliner, R.S. 1939. The prevention of carotene absorption by liquid petrolatum. *J.A.M.A.*113:1785.

76. Damrau, F. 1961. The value of bentonite for diarrhea. *Medical Annals District Columbia* 30 (6) pp. 326-28.

77. Darsee, J.R., Heymsfield, S.B. 1981. Decreased myocardial taurine levels. *N.E.J.M.* 304:129.

78. Davies, I.J. 1972. *The Clinical Significance of the Essential Biological Metals.* Charles C. Thomas, Publisher.

79. Davies, S., Stewart, A. 1987. *Nutritional Medicine.* Pan Books, London.

80. Dawson-Hughes, B., Seligson, F.H., Hughes, V.A. 1986. Effects of calcium carbonate and hydroxyapatite on zinc and iron retention in postmenopausal women. *Am. J. Clin. Nutr.* 44:83-88.

81. Dean, R., Cheeseman, K. 1987. Vitamin E protects against free radical damage in lipid environments. *Bioc. Biop. R.* 148:1277-82.

82. Diamond, H. and Diamond, M. 1985. *Fit for Life.* Warner Books, Inc. New York.

83. Dillard, C.J., et al. 1978. Effects of exercise, vitamin E, and ozone on pulmonary function and lipid peroxidation. *J. Appl. Physiol.* 45:927-32.

84. DiLuzio, N.R. 1973. Antioxidants, lipid peroxidation, and chemical-induced liver injury. *Fed. Proc.* 32:1875-81.

85. DiMagno, E.P., et al. 1977. Fate of orally ingested enzymes in pancreatic insufficiency. *N.E.J.M.* 296(23): 1318-22.

86. DiPerna, P. 1984. Leukemia strikes a small town. *New York Times Magazine*, pp. 100-08.

87. Donahue, R.P., et al. 1987. Central obesity and coronary heart disease in men. *Lancet* 1:821.

88. Dormandy, T.L. 1978. Free radical oxidation and antioxidants. *Lancet* 1:647-50.

89. Drasar, B.S., Hill, M.J. 1972. Intestinal bacteria and cancer. *Amer. J. Clin. Nutr.* 25:1399-1404.

90. Dreizen, S. 1979. Nutrition and the immune response—a review. *Int. J.Vit. Nutr. Res.* 49:220.

91. Droull, J. 1982. *Drinking Water and Health.* Vol. 4. National Academy of Sciences Press, Washington, D.C.

92. Duke, J.A. 1985. *Handbook of Medicinal Herbs.* CRC Press, Boca Raton, FL.

93. Eaton, S., Konner, M. 1985. Paleolithic nutrition. *N.E.J.M.* 312(5) Jan. 31.

94. Edington, J., Geekie, M., Charter, R., et al. 1987. Effect of dietary cholesterol on plasma cholesterol concentration in subjects following reduced fat, high fiber diet. *Br. Med. J.* 294:333-36.

95. Elwood, P.C., et al. 1984. Greater contribution to blood lead from water than from air. *Nature* 310:138-40.

96. Ensminger, A.H., et al. 1983. *Foods and Nutrition Encyclopedia.* Vol. 1&2. Pergus Press, Clovis, CA.

97. Fannelli, O. 1978. Carnitine and acetyle-carnitine, natural substances endowed with interesting pharmacological properties. *Life Sci.* 23:2563-70.

98. Farber, E. 1981. Chemical carcinogenesis. *N.E.J.M.* 305:1379.

99. Fernandes, K.M., Shahani, M.A. 1987. Therapeutic role of dietary lactobacilli and lactobacillic fermented dairy products. *F.E.M.S. Micro. Rev.* (Sept.) 46:343-56.

100. Florence, T.M. 1984. Cancer and aging: the free radical connection. *Int. Clin. Nutr. Rev.* 4 (1) pp 6-19.

101. Foldi, M. 1972. Vitamin P and Lymphatics. *Angiologica* 9(3):375-89.

102. Folkers, K., Yamamura, Y. (eds). 1986. *Biomedical and Clinical Applications of Coenzyme Q-10.* Bantam Books.

103. Fox, M. 1984. *Healthy Water for a Longer Life.* Healthy Water Research Institute. Las Vegas, Nevada.

104. Francis, A., Shetty, T., Bhattach, R. 1988. Modifying role of dietary factors on the mutagenicity of aflatoxin B1: in vitro effects of trace minerals. *Mutat. Res.* 199:85-93.

105. Freeman, B.A., Crapo, J.D. 1982. Biology of disease: free radicals and tissue injury. *Lab. Invest.* 47:412-426.

106. Fritz, I.B. 1963. Carnitine and its role in fatty acid metabolism. *Adv. Lipid Res.* 1:285-334.

107. Frost, D.V., Lish, P.M. 1975. Selenium in biology. *Ann. Rev. Pharm.* 75(15): 259-84.

108. Fujita, T., et al. 1987. Effects of increased adrenomedullary activity and taurine in patients with borderline hypertension. *Circulation* 75:525.

109. Fujisawa, K., Suzuki, H., et al. 1984. Therapeutic effects of liver hydrolysate preparation on chronic hepatitis—a double blind, controlled study. *Asian Med. J.* 26:497-526.

110. Fulder, S.J. 1981. Ginseng and the hypothalamic-pituitary control of stress. *Am. J. Chin. Med.* 9:112-8.

111. Gettis, A. 1987. Serendipity and food sensitivity: a case study. *Headache Journal* 27:73-75.

112. Gibson, G.E, et al. 1988. Reduced activities of thiamine-dependent enzymes in the brains and peripheral tissues of patients with Alzheimer's disease. *Archives of Neurology* 45:836-40.

113. Glavind, L., Zeuner, E. 1986. The effectiveness of a rotary electric toothbrush on oral cleanliness in adults. *J. Clin. Periodont.* 13(2):135-38.

114. Goldberg, I.K. 1980. L-tyrosine in depression. *Lancet* 2:364.

115. Goldman, I.S., Kantrowitz, N.E. 1982. Cardiomyopathy associated with selenium deficiency. *N.E.J.M.* 305:701.

116. Goldstein, G.W. 1977. Lead encephalopathy: the significance of lead inhibition of calcium uptake by brain mitochondria. *Brain Res.* (Netherlands) 136(1):185-188.

117. Grant, E.C. 1979. Food allergies and migraine. *Lancet* 5:966.

118. Griffith, R., et al. 1987. Success of L-lysine therapy in frequently recurrent herpes simplex infection. *Dermatolog.* 175:183-90.

119. Grundy, S., Florentin, L., Nix, D., et al. 1988. Comparison of monounsaturated fatty acids and carbohydrates for reducing raised levels of plasma cholesterol in man. *Am. J. Clin. Nutr.* 47:966-69.

120. Gupta, S., Agarwal, L.B., Epstein, G., et al. 1980. Panax: a new mitogen and interferon producer. *Clin. Res.* 28:504A.

121. Gutteridge, J.M., et al. 1982. Superoxide-dependent formation of hydroxyl radicals and lipid peroxidation in the presence of iron salts. *Biochem. J.* 206:605-09.

122. Hackney, J.D., et al. 1975. Experimental studies on human health effects of air pollutants. II *Ozone Arch. Envir. Hlth* 30:379-84.

276   EAT RIGHT OR DIE YOUNG

123. Hall, K. 1976. Allergy of the nervous system: a review. *Ann. Allergy* 36:49.

124. Halliwell, B., Gutteridge, J.M.C. 1984. Lipid peroxidation, oxygen radicals, cell damage, and antioxidant therapy. *Lancet* 1396-97.

125. Harris, J.B., et al. 1967. Lipoic acid: essential cofactor for gastric secretion. *Fed. Proc.* 26:273.

126. Havsteen, B. 1983. Flavonoids, a class of natural products of high pharmacological potency. *Biochem. Pharm.* 32:1141-8.

127. Heimburger, D., et al. 1987. Improvement in bronchial squamous metaplasia in smoker treated with folate and B-12. *Am. J. Clin. Nutr.* 45:866.

128. Hicks, J.T. 1964. Treatment of fatigue in general practice: a double-blind study. *Clin. Med. J.* pp. 85-90.

129. Hikino, H., Kiso, Y., Wagner, H., et al. 1984. Antihepatotoxic actions of flavonolignans from Silybum marianum fruits. *Planta Medica* 50:248.

130. Hill, M.J., Drasar, B.S., Aries, V., et al. 1971. Bacteria and the etiology of cancer of the large bowel. *Lancet* 1:95-100.

131. Hirayama, S., Kishikawa, H., Kume, T., et al. 1978. Therapeutic effect of liver hydrolysate on experimental liver cirrhosis. *Nisshin Igaku* 45:528-33.

132. Hollander, D., Tarnawski, H. 1985. Aging-associated increase in intestinal absorption of macromolecules. *Gerontology* 31:133-37.

133. Hollman, J., et al. 1983. Coronary artery spasm at site of previous angioplasty. *J. Amer. Coll. Card.* 2:1039-1045.

134. Horrobin, D.F., Manku, M.S. 1983. Essential fatty acids in clinical medicine. *Nutrition and Health* 2:127-34.

135. Horwitt, M.K. 1980. Relative biological values of D-alpha-tocopheryl acetate and all-rac-A tocopheryl acetate in man. *Am. J. Clin. Nutr.* 33:1856-1860.

136. Horwitt, M.K. 1980. Therapeutic uses of vitamin E in medicine. *Nutr. Rev.* 38(3).

137. Hoyumpa, A.M. 1983. Alcohol and thiamine metabolism. *Alcoholism: Clinical and Experimental Research* 7(1).

138. Isaacs, J.P., Lamb, B.S. 1974. Trace metals, vitamins, and hormones in ten-year treatment of coronary atherosclerotic heart disease. *Texas Heart Institute Symposium* Feb. 21.

139. Isselbacher, K.J. 1977. Metabolic and hepatic effect of alcohol. *N.E.J.M.* March 17, 296(11).

140. Jamal, G.A., Carmichael, H., Weir, A.I. 1986. Gamma-linolenic acid in diabetic neuropathy. *Lancet* May 10, letter to the editor.

141. Jacques, P., et al. 1987. Vitamin intake and senile cataract. *J. Am. Col. Nutr.* 6:435.

142. Jayaraj, A.P., Tovey, F.I., Clark, C.G. 1980. Possible dietary protective factors in relation to the distribution of duodenal ulcer in India and Bangladesh. *Gut* 21:1068-76.

143. Jensen, B. 1987. *Chlorella: Gem of the Orient.* Bernard Jensen Publisher, Escondido, CA.

144. Johns, D.R. 1986. Migraine provoked by aspartame. *N.E.J.M.* 315:456.

145. Johnson, F.C. 1979. The antioxidant vitamins. *CRC Crit. Rev. Food Sci. Nutr.* 11:217-309.

146.. Jones, A.V., Shorhouse, M., McLaughlan, P., et. al. 1982. Food intolerance: a major factor in the pathogenesis of irritable bowel syndrome. *Lancet* Nov. 20.

147. Jones, L.A.O., Gould, J.H. 1980. Elemental content of predigested liquid protein products. *Amer. J. Clin. Nutr.* 33:2545.

148. Jones, M.H. 1984. *The Allergy Self-Help Cookbook.* Rodale Press, Inc., Emmanus, Penn.

149. Kabacoff, B.L., et. al. 1963. Absorption of chymotrypsin from the intestinal tract. *Nature* 199:815.

150. Kagawa, K., et. al. 1986. Garlic extract inhibits the enhanced peroxidation and production of lipids in carbon tetrachloride-induced liver injury. *Jap. J. Pharm.* 42:19.

151. Kamm, J.J., Dashman, T., Connely., A., et. al. 1975. Effect of ascorbic acid on amine nitrite toxicity. *Ann. New York Acad. Sci.* 258:169-74.

152. Kamm, J.J., Dashman, T., Newmark, H., et. al. 1977. Inhibition of amine nitrite hepatotoxicity by alpha-tocopherol. *Toxicol. Appl. Pharm.* 41:575-83.

153. Kandil, O.M., et. al. 1987. Garlic and the immune system in humans: its effect on natural killer cells. *Fed. Proc.* 46:441.

154. Kannel, W.B., Pearson, G., McNamara, M. 1969. Obesity as a force of morbidity and mortality. F.P. Herald (ed). *Adolescent Nutrition and Growth.*

155. Karkkainen, P., et. al. 1986. Alcohol intake correlated with serum trace elements. *Alc. Alcohol* 23:279-82.

156. Kaul, T.N., Middleton, E., Ogra, P.L. 1985. Anti-viral effect of flavonoids on human viruses. *J. Med. Virol.* 15:71-9.

157. Kelsay, J.L., et. al. 1979. Effect of fiber from fruits and vegetables on metabolic responses of human subjects. *Am. J. Clin. Nutr.* 32:1876.

158. Kendler, B. 1987. Garlic and onion: a review of their relationship to cardiovascular disease. *Prev. Med.* 16:670-85.

159. Kennedy, M.J., Volz, P.A. 1985. Ecology of candida albicans gut colonization: inhibition of candida adhesion, colonization, and dissemination from the gastrointestinal tract by bacterial antagonism. *Infection and Immunity* 49(3):654-63.

160. Kikuchi, Y., Koyama, T. 1983. Cholesterol-induced impairment in red cell deformability and its improvement by vitamin E. *Clin. Hemorh.* 3:375.

161. Kiso, Y., Suzuki, Y., Watanabe, N., et. al. 1983. Antihepatotoxic principles of Curcuma longa rhizomes. *Planta Medica* 49:185-7.

162. Kligman, A., Mills, O., Leyden, J., et. al. 1981. Oral vitamin A in acne vulgaris. *Int. J. Derm.* 20:278-85.

163. Knapp, H.R., Reilly, I., Alessandrini, P., et. al. 1986. In vivo indexes of platelet and vascular function during fish-oil administration in patients with atherosclerosis. *N.E.J.M.* Apr. 10, pp. 937-42.

164. Kok, F.J., et. al. 1989. Decreased selenium levels in acute myocardial infarction. *J.A.M.A.* 261(8):1161-64.

165. Kondoh, M., Ohe, M., Akifumi, O., et. al. 1984. Effect of sodium saccharin on rat pancreatic enzyme secretion. *J. Nutr. Sci. Vitaminol.* 30:569-76.

166. Konishi, F., et. al. 1985. Anti-tumor effect induced by a hot water extract of chlorella vulgaris (CE): resistence to meth-A tumor growth mediated by CE-induced polymorphonuclear leukocytes. *Cancer Immunol. Immunother.* 19:73-78.

167. Kopaladze, R.A., Turova, N.F. 1985. Correction of impaired oxygen supply with antioxidants. *Izv. Akad. Gruz. SSR. Ser. Biol.* 11:324-9.

168. Kornhauser, A., et. al. 1986. Protective effects of beta carotene against psoralen toxicity: relevance to protection against carcinogenesis. *Anti-Mutagenesis and Anticarcinogenesis Mechanisms.* Plenum Press, New York.

169. Korovka, L.S. 1976. Ascorbic acid content in wild growing edible plants of Komi-Permiak National Okrug, USSR. *Vopr. Pitan.* (6):76-77.

170. Korpela, H., Kumpulainen, J.T., Sotaniemi, E.A. 1985. The role of selenium deficiency in the pathogenesis of alcoholic liver disease. *Nutrition Research,* Suppl. 1; pp. 424-25. Pergamon Press, LTD.

171. Krause, M.V., Mahan, L.K. 1984. *Food, Nutrition, and Diet Therapy.* W.B. Sanders Co., Philadelphia, Penn.

172. Krinsky, N., et. al. 1982. Interaction of oxygen and oxy-radicals with carotenoids. *J. Can. Res. Clin. Onco.* 69:205.

173. Kromhout, D., Coulander, C. 1982. Dietary fiber and 10 year mortality from coronary heart disease, cancer and all causes. *Lancet* Sept. 4:518.

174. Kuhnau, J., 1976. The flavonoids: a class of semi-essential food components: their role in human nutrition. *Wld Rev. Diet* 24:117-91.

175. Kuller, L. 1969. Sudden death in atherosclerotic heart disease. The case for preventive medicine. *Amer. J. Card.* 24:617.

176. Lahman, S. 1970. Studies on placental transfer: trichloroethylene. *Ind. Med.* 39:46-9.

177. Langer, S.E., Scheer, J.F. 1984. *Solved: The Riddle of Illness.* Keats Publishing, Inc., New Canaan, Conn.

178. Langsjoen, P.H., Vadhanavikit, S., Folkers, K. 1985. Response of patients in classes III and IV of cardiomyopathy to therapy in a blind and crossover trial with coenzyme Q-10. *Proc. Natl. Acad. Sci.* 82:4240.

179. Lau, B.H.S., et. al. 1987. Effect of an odor-modified garlic preparation on blood lipids. *Nutr. Res.* 7:139.

180. Lau, B.H.S., et. al. 1983. Allium sativum (garlic) and atherosclerosis: a review. *Nutr. Res.* 3:119.

181. Laurent, J., Rostoker, R., Robeva, C., et. al. 1987. Is adult idiopathic nephrotic syndrome food allergy? value of oligoantigenic diets. *Nephron* (Sept.) 47:7-11.

182. Lawson, M., Bunker, V., Clayton, B., et. al. 1987. The effect of dietary fibre on apparent absorption of zinc, copper, iron and manganese in the elderly. *P. Nutr. Soc.* 46:53A.

183. LeGrady, D., et. al. 1987. Coffee consumption and mortality in the Chicago Western Electric Company. *Am. J. Epidem.* 126:803-812.

184. Lessof, M.H. (ed.) 1983. *Clinical Reactions to Foods.* John Wiley & Sons, Chichester.

185. Levine, S.A., Kidd, P.M. 1987. *Antioxidant Adaptation: Its Role in Free Radical Pathology.* Biocurrents Division, Allergy Res. Group, Publisher.

186. Levine, S.A., Kidd, P.A. 1985. Biochemical pathologies initiated by free radical oxidant compounds in the etiology of food hypersensitivity disease. *Int. Clin. Nutr. Rev.* 5(1):5-23.

187. Lindenbaum, J., Healton, E., Savage, D., et. al. 1988. Neuropsychiatric disorders caused by cobalamin deficiency in the absence of anemia or macrocytosis. *N.E.J.M.* 318:1720-28.

188. Littarru, G.P., Ho, L., Folkers, K. 1972. Deficiency of coenzyme Q-10 in human heart disease. Part II. *Internat. J. Vit. Res.* 42:413.

189. Lonsdale, D. 1987. Thiamine and its fat soluble derivatives as therapeutic agents. *Int. Clin. Nutr. Rev.* 7(3):114-25

190. Maebashi, M. 1978. Lipid-lowering effect of carnitine in patients with type IV hyperlipoproteinaemia. *Lancet* 1:805.

191. Malkinson, F. 1964. Permeability of the stratum corneum. In: W. Montagna, W.E. Lobit, Jr. (eds): *The Epidermis.* Academic Press. New York.

192. Mallos, T. 1979. *The Complete Middle East Cookbook.* McGraw-Hill, New York.

193. Massey, L., et. al. 1988. Acute effects of dietary caffeine and aspirin on urinary mineral excretion in pre- and postmenopausal women. *Nutr. Res.* 845-51.

194. Marshall, A.W., et al. 1982. Treatment of alcohol-related liver disease with thioctic acid: a six month randomized double-blind trial. *Gut* 23:1088-93.

195. McClain, C.J., Su, L. 1983. Zinc deficiency in the alcoholic: a review. *Alcoholism: Clinical and Experimental Research* 7(1).

196. McLennan, P., Abeywardena, M., Charnock, J. 1988. Dietary fish oil prevents ventricular fibrillation following coronary artery occlusion and reperfusion. *Am. Heart J.* 116:709-17.

197. Meck, W., Church, R. 1987. Nutrients that modify the speed of internal clock and memory storage processes. *Behav. Neuro.* 101:465-75.

198. Mengel, C.E. 1968. Rancidity of the red cell. Peroxidation of red cell lipid. *Amer. J. Sci.* June 255:341-45.

199. Michaelson, G., Juhlin, L., Vahlquist, A. 1977. Effects of oral zinc and vitamin A in acne. *Arch. Derm.* 113:31-6.

200. Michaelson, G., Vahiquist, A., Juhlin, L. 1977. Serum zinc and retinol binding-protein in acne. *Br. J. Derm.* 96:283-6.

201. Middleton, E. 1984. The flavonoids. trends in pharmaceutical science. *Science* 5:335-8.

202. Miller, D.S., Parsonage, S. 1975. Resistance to slimming: adaptation or illusion? *Lancet* Apr. 5, p. 773.

203. Miller, J.D. 1982. The new pollution: ground water contamination. *Environment* 24:8.

204. Misiewicz, G. 1972. Gastrointestinal manifestations of stress and the psychopathic personality. *Medicine* 3:183-88.

205. Mock, D., Johnson, S., Holman, R. 1988. Effects of biotin deficiency on serum fatty acid composition: evidence for abnormalities in humans. *J. Nutr.* 118:342-48.

206. Monro, J., Brostoff, J. 1980. Food allergy in migraine. *Lancet* July 5:1014

207. Morley, J.E. 1982. Food peptides— a new class of hormones? *J.A.M.A.* 17:2379-80.

208. Moses, H.A. 1979. Trace elements: an association with cardiovascular diseases and hypertension: *J. Nat'l. Med. Assoc.* 71(3):227-28.

209. Mueller, L.J., et. al. 1987. Rotary electric toothbrushing — clinical effects on the presence of gingivitis and supragingival dental plaque. *Dental Hygiene* 61(12):546-50.

210. Mussalo-Rauhamaa, H., et. al. 1987. Decreased serum selenium and magnesium levels in drunkenness arrestees. *Drug Al. Dep.* 20:95-103.

211. Nakazono, K. 1985. Active oxygen and factors scavenging it in synovial fluid in rheumatoid arthritis. *Nigata Igakkai Zasshi* 99:489-501.

212. Nely, J.R., Morgen, H.E. 1974. Relationships between carbohydrates and lipid metabolism and the energy balance of the heart muscle. *Ann. Rev. Physical.* 36: 413-460.

213. Niki, E., Tsuchiya, J., Yoshikawa, Y., et al. 1986. Oxidation of lipids. XIII. Antioxidant activities of alpha-, beta-, gamma-, and delta-tocopherols. *Bull. Chem. Soc. Jpn* 59:497-501.

214. Novi, A.M., Flokke, R. Stukenkemper, M. 1982. Glutathione and aflatoxin B1-induced liver tumors: requirement for an intact glutathione molecule for regression of malignancy. In R. Baserga (ed). Cell proliferation, Cancer, and Cancer Therapy: a conference in honor of Ann Goldfeder. *New York Academy of Sciences Annals* 397:62-71.

215. Oelgetz, A.W., et al. 1935. The treatment of food allergy and indigestion of pancreatic origin with pancreatic enzymes. *Amer. J. Dig. Dis. Nutr.* 2:422-26.

216. Oelgetz, A.W., et al. 1939. Pancreatic enzymes and food allergy. *Med. Rec.* 150:276-79.

217. Offenbacher, E., Stunyer, F. 1980. Beneficial effect of chromium-rich yeast on glucose tolerance and blood lipids in elderly patients. *Diabetes* 29:919-25.

218. Opie, L.H. 1977. Role of carnitine in fatty acid metabolism of normal and ischemic myocardium. *Am. Heart J.* 3:375.

219. Oram J.F., Wenger, J.I., Neely, J.R. 1975. Regulation of long chain fatty acid activation in the heart muscle. *J. Biol. Chem.* 250:73-78.

220. Orengo, I., et al. 1988. The influence of dietary menhaden oil upon photocarcinogenesis. *Clin. Res.* 36:85A.

221. Orengo, I., Black, H., Kettler, A., et al. 1988. Influence of dietary menhaden oil upon carcinogenesis and related responses to UV-radiation. (meeting abstract). *J. Inv. Derm.* 90:594.

222. Pauling, L. 1986. *How to Live Longer and Feel Better.* W.H. Freeman and Co. New York.

223. Pereira, M.A., et al. 1982. Trihalomethanes as inhibitors and promoters of carcinogenesis. *Envir. Hlth Persp.* 46:151-56.

224. Petersdorf, R. (ed). 1983. *Harrison's Principles of Internal Medicine.* 10th ed. McGraw Hill, New York.

225. Peticone, F., et al. 1988. Protective magnesium treatment in ischemic dilated cardiomyopathy (meeting abstract). *J. Am. Col. Nutr.* 7:403.

226. Pothier, L., et al. 1987. Plasma selenium levels in patients with advanced upper gastrointestinal cancer. *Cancer* 60:2251-2260.

227. Prasad, K.N. 1982. Effects of tocopherol on morhological alterations and growth inhibition in melanoma cells in culture. *Cancer Res.* 42:550.

228. Prasad, K.M., Bhola, N.R. 1984. Nutrition and cancer. In *Yearbook of Nutritional Medicine*, J. Bland, (ed). 1:178-89.

229. Pryor, W.A. (ed). 1976. *Free Radicals in Biology.* Vol. 1-3. Academic Press, New York.

230. Puddey, I.B. 1987. Regular alcohol use raises blood pressure in treated hypertensive subjects. *Lancet* 10:647-651.

231. Pye, V.I., Patrick, R. 1983. Ground water contamination in the United States. *Science* 221:713-18.

232. Randi, A., et al. 1987. Orally administered vitamin B-6 prolongs the bleeding time and inhibits platelet aggregation in human volunteers. *Thromb. Haem.* 58:176.

232. Reading, C.M., Meillon, R.S. 1988. *The Family Tree Connection.* Keats Publishing, Inc. New Canaan, Conn.

233. Rebouche, C.J., Engel, A.G. 1980. Tissue distribution of carnitine biosynthetic enzymes in man. *Biochem. Biophys. Acta.* 630:22-29.

234. Reed, L.J. 1953. Metabolic functions of thiamin and lipoic acid. *Physical Rev.* 33:544-59.

235. Reid, K., et al. 1987. Double-blind study of yohimbine in treatment of psychogenic impotence. *Lancet* 2:241.

236. Reiser, S., et al. 1987. Effect of copper intake on blood cholesterol and its lipoprotein distribution in men. *Nutr. Rep. In.* 36:641-49.

237. Reiter, L., et al. 1987. Vitamin B-12 and folate intakes and plasma levels of black adolescent females. *J. Am. Diet. Assoc.* 87.

238. Resnik, L. 1987. Interrelation of calcium and magnesium with renin-sodium factors in essential hypertension. *J. Am. Coll. Nutr.* 6:62-63.

239. Riales, R., Albrink, M. 1981. Effects of chromium chloride supplementation on the glucose tolerance and serum lipids, including HDL, in adult men. *Am. J. Clin. Nutr.* 34:2670-8.

240. Rice, S.L., Eiten Miller, R.R., Koehler, P.E. 1976. Biologically active amines in food: a review. *J. Milk. Food Technol.* 39(5):353-8.

241. Robson, J.R.K., et al. 1977. Metabolic response to food. *Lancet* Dec. 24 & 31, p. 1267.

242. Roe, D.A. 1983. *Drug-Induced Nutritional Deficiences.* A.V.I., Westport, Conn.

243. Rogers, S. 1985. Sugar and health. *Lancet* Feb. 23.

244. Rosenberg, E., Belew, P. 1982. Microbial factors in psoriasis. *Arch. Derm.* 118:1434-44.

245. Rosenberg, L., et al. 1982. Breast cancer and alcoholic beverage consumption. *Lancet* Jan 30:267.

246. Rossi, C.S., Siliprandi, N. 1982. Effect of carnitine on serum HDL cholesterol: report of two cases. *John Hopkins Med. J.* 150:51-54.

247. Rowe, N.A., Gorlin, R.J. 1959. The effect of vitamin A deficiency upon experimental oral carcinogenesis. *J. Dent. Res. Jan-Feb,* pp. 72-83.

248. Ruddel H., et al. 1987. Effect of magnesium supplementation in patients with labile hypertension. *J. Amer. Coll. Nutr.* 6:445.

249. Saffiotti, J., Montesano, R., Sellakumar, D.V.M., et al. 1967. Experimental cancer of the lung. Inhibition by vitamin A of induction of tracheobronchial squamous metaplasia. *Cancer* May, pp. 857-63.

250. Sakula, A., et al. 1980. Vitamin A and cancer. *Lancet* 2:1029.

251. Salonen, J., et al. 1988. Relationship of serum selenium and antioxidants to plasma lipoproteins, platelet aggregability and prevalent ischaemic heart disease in Eastern Finnish men. *Atherosclerosis* 70:155-60.

252. Salmi, H.A., Sarna, S. 1982. Effect of silymarin on chemical, functional, and morphological alterations of liver. A double-blind controlled study. *Scand. J. Gastroenterol.* 17:517-21.

253. Samuni, A., et al. 1981. Unusual oxygen-induced sensitization of the biological damage due to superoxide radicals. *J. Biol. Chem.* 256:12632.

254. Sandhu, D.K., Warraich, M.K., Singh, S. 1980. Sensitivity of yeasts isolated from cases of vaginitis to aqueous extract of garlic. *Mykosen* 23(12):3169-73.

255. Sandine, W.E. 1979. Roles of lactobacillus in test intestinal tract. *Journal of Food Protection* 42:259-62.

256. Scholar, E., et al. 1988. Effects of diets enriched in cabbage and collards on metastasis of BALB/c mammary carcinoma (meeting abstract). *P. Am. Assoc. Ca.* 29:149.

257. Schrauzer, G.N. 1976. Selenium and cancer: a review. *Bioinorganic Chemistry* 5:275.

258. Schrauzer, G.N. 1977. Cancer mortality correlation studies III. Statistical associations with dietary selenium intakes. *Bioinorganic Chemistry* 7:23

259. Schrauzer, G.N., White, D.A. 1978. Selenium in human nutrition: dietary intakes and effects of supplementation. *Bioinorganic Chemistry* 8:303-18.

260. Schroeder, H.A. 1973. *The Trace Elements and Man.* Devin-Adair Co., Old Greenwich, Conn.

261. Schroeder, H.A. 1974. *The Poisons Around Us.* Indiana Univ. Press, London.

262. Schwarz, K.S. 1970. The cellular mechanisms of vitamin E action: direct and indirect effects of alpha-tocopherol on mitochondrial respiration. *Ann. N.Y. Acad. Sci.*

263. Scragg, R., et al. 1982. Birth defects in household water supply. Epidemiological studies in the mount Gambier region of South Australia. *Med. J. Austr.* 2:577-79.

264. Scriver, C.R., Rosenberg, L.E. 1973. Amino acid metabolism and its disorders. Alex Schaffer (ed). *Major Problems in Clinical Pediatrics.* W.B. Saunders Co., Philadelphia.

265. Seelig, M.S., Heggtveit, H.A. 1974. Magnesium interrelationships in ischemic heart disease: a review. *Am. J. Clin. Nutr.* 27:59.

266. Seiss, W., Roth, P.P., Scherer, B.C., et al. 1980. Platelet membrane fatty acids, platelet aggregation and thromboxane formation during mackerel diet. *Lancet* March pp.441-44.

267. Shamberger, R.J. 1976. Selenium in health and disease. *Proc. Symp. Selen. Tell. Envir.* Industrial Health Foundation, Inc. Pittsburgh, Penn.

268. Shariff, R., et al. 1988. Vitamin E supplementation in smokers. *Clin. Res.* 36:A770.

269. Shaw, D.M., et al. 1984. Senile dementia and nutrition. (Letter to the editor). *Brit. Med. J.* 288:792-93.

270. Shaw, J.H. 1987. Causes and control of dental caries. *N.E.J.M.* 317:996.

271. Shaw, S., Lieber, C.S. 1983. Plasma amino acids in the alcoholic: nutritional aspects. *Alcoholism: Clinical and Experimental Research* 7(1).

272. Siccardi, A., Fortunato, A., Marconi, M., et al. 1981. Defective bactericidal reaction by the alternative pathway of complement in atopic patients. *Infect. Immun.* 33:701-3.

273. Snook, J.T., Palmquist, D.L., et al. 1983. Selenium status of a rural (predominately Amish) community living in a low-selenium area. *Am. J. Clin. Nutr.* 38:620.

274. Sohler, A., Kruesi, M., Pfeiffer, C.C. 1977. Blood lead levels in psychiatric outpatients reduced by zinc and vitamin C. *J. Orthomol. Psy.* 6(3):272-276.

275. Solinan, M.A., Fahmy, S.A., et al. 1970. Liver cell regeneration in prophylaxis and treatment of carbon tetrachloride hepatotoxicity. *J. Egypt. Med. Assoc.* 53(3):214-22.

276. Spallholz, J.E. 1981. Anti-inflammatory, immunological, and carcinostatic attributes of selenium in experimental animals. *Adv. Exp. Med. Biol.* 135:43-61.

277. Stampfer, M.J., Hennekens, C.H. 1982. Carotene, carrots, and white blood cells. *Lancet* Sept. 11:615.

278. Steenblock, D. 1987. *Chlorella: Natural Medicinal Algae.* Aging Research Institute, El Toro, Calif.

279. Stevens, R., et al. 1988. Body iron stores and the risk of cancer. *Am. J. Clin. Nutr.* 319:1047-52.

280. Stevenson, D. 1979. Food allergies and migraine. *Lancet* July 14:103.

281. Stewart, R., Dodd, H. 1964. Absorption of carbon tetrachloride, trichloroethylene, tetrachloroethylene, methylene chloride, and 1, 1, 1-trichloroethane through human skin. *Ind. Hyg. J.* Sept. - Oct. pp. 439-46.

282. Suda, D., et al. 1986. Inhibition of experimental oral carcinogenesis by topical beta carotene. *Carcinogenesis* 7:711

283. Suekawa, M., Ishige, A., Yuasa, K., et al. 1984. Pharmacological studies on ginger. I. Pharmacological actions of pungent constituents, (6)-gingerol and (6)-shogaol. *J. Pharm. Dyn.* 7:836-48.

284. Sugino, K., Kiyohiko, D., Yamoda, K., et al. 1987. The role of lipid peroxidation in endotoxin-induced hepatic damage and the protective effect of antioxidants. *Surgery* June 1; Vol. 6.

285. Sugiyama, S., Kitazawa, M., Ozawa, K., et al. 1980. Antioxidative effect of coenzyme Q-10. *Experiontia* 36:1002.

286. Sullivan, J.L. 1981. Iron and the sex difference in heart diesease risk. *Lancet* June 13, p. 1239.

287. Sullivan, J.L. 1983. Vegetarianism, ischemic heart disease, and iron. (letter to the editor). *Am. J. Clin. Nutr.* 37:882-86.

288. Suzuki, Y., Kamikawa, T., Yamazaki, N. 1980. Protective effects of l-carnitine on ischemic heart. *Carnitine Biosynthesis, Metabolism, and Functions.* Academic Press, pp. 341-52.

289. Swain, A., Truswell, A.S., Loblay, R.H. 1984. Adverse reactions to food. *Food Technology in Australia.* 36(10): 467-71.

290. Swain, A., Dutton, S.P., Truswell, A.S. 1985. Salicylates in foods. *J. Amer. Diet. Assoc.* 85(8):950-60.

291. Szejnwald-Brown, H., Bishop, D.R., Rowan, C.A. 1984. The role of skin absorption as a route of exposure for volatile organic compounds (VOCs) in drinking water. *Amer. J. Pub. Hlth* 74(S):479-83.

292. Tanaka, K. 1981. New light on biotin deficiency. *N.E.J.M.* 304:839-40.

293. Tappel, A.L. 1973. Lipid peroxidation damage to cell components. *Fed. Proc.* 32:1870-74.

294. Tappel, A.L. 1980. On antioxidant nutrients: how they may protect you from smog and other environmental pollutants and some aging reactions. *Executive Health Magazine.*

295. Tappel, A.L. 1980. Measurement of and protection from in vivo lipid peroxidation. W.W. Pryor (ed). *Free Radicals in Biology* 4:2-47.

296. Tarayre, J.P., Lauressergies, H., et al. 1977. Advantages of a combination of proteolytic enzymes, flavonoids, and ascorbic acid in comparison with non-steroidal anti-inflammatory agents. *Arznein-Forsch. Drug Res.* 27(1):1144.

297. Tengroth, B., Ammitzboll, T. 1984. Changes in the content and composition of collagen in the glaucomatous eye — basis for a new hypothesis for the genesis of chronic open angle glaucoma. *Acta. Opthamol.* 62:999-1008.

298. Thomsen, M., et al. 1978. Improved pacing tolerance of the ischemic human myocardium after administration of carnitine. *Am. J. Cardiol.* 43:304.

299. Towns, S.J., Mellis, C.M. 1984. Role of acetyl salicylic acid and sodium metabisulphite in chronic childhood asthma. *Pediatrics* 73(5):631-7.

300. Trivellato, M., et al. 1984. Carnitine deficiency as the possible etiology of idiopathic mitral valve prolapse: case study with speculative annotation. *Texas Heart Institute Journal* 11(4):370

301. Tuchweber, B., Trost, W., Salas, M., et al. 1976. Prevention of praseodymium-induced hepatotoxicity by silybin. *Toxicol. Appl. Pharmacol.* 38:559-70.

302. Ulrey, D.E. 1976. Selenium in animal nutrition: health implication. *Proc. Symp. Selen. Tell. Envr.* Industrial Health Foundation Inc., Pittsburgh, Penn.

303. Upadhyay, M.P., Manadhar, K.L., Shrestha, R.B. 1980. Anti-fungal activity of garlic against fungi isolated from human eyes. *J. Gen. Appl. Microbiol.* 26(6):421-24.

304. Vahouny, G., Kritchevsky, D. 1982. *Dietary Fiber in Health and Disease.* Plenem Press, New York.

305. Vander, A.J. 1981. *Nutrition, Stress and Toxic Chemicals.* University of Michigan Press, Ann Arbor, Mich.

306. Vanderhoek, J.Y., Makheja, A.H., Bailey, J.M. 1980. Inhibition of fatty-acid oxygenases by onion and garlic oils evidence for the mechanism by which these oils inhibit platelet aggregation. *Biochem. Pharmacol.* 29(23):3169-73.

307. Wald, N., et al. 1988. Serum beta-carotene and subsequent risk of cancer: results from the BUPA study. *Br. J. Canc.* 57:428-33.

308. Waldbott, G.L. 1978. *Health Effects of Environmental Pollutants.* 2nd ed. C.V.Mosby Co., St. Louis.

309. Wald, N., et al. 1987. Serum vitamin E and subsequent risk of cancer. *Br. J. Canc.* 56:69-72.

310. Walker, W.A. 1981. *Intestinal Transport of Macromolecules. Physiology of the Gastrointestinal Tract.* L.R. Johnson (ed). Raven Press, New York.

311. Walker, W.A. 1982. Mechanisms of antigen handling by the gut. *Clinics in Immunology and Allergy* 2(1):15-35.

312. Wang, L.F., Lin, J.K., Tung, Y.C. 1979. Protective effect of chlorella on hepatic damage induced by ethionine in rats. *J. Formosan Med. Assoc.* 78:1010-19.

313. Ward, R., Peters, D.P. 1987. Nutritional and vitamin E status of alcohol abusers with and without chronic skeletal muscle myopathy. *Alc. Alcohol* 22:A6.

314. Watson, R., Leonard, T. 1986. Selenium and vitamins A, E, and C: nutrients with cancer prevention properties. *J. Am. Diet. Assoc.* 86:505-10.

315. Webster, P., Dyckner, T. 1987. Magnesium and hypertension. *J. Am. Coll. Nutr.* 6:321-8.

316. Webster, R., Maibach, H. 1977. Percutaneous absorption in man and animal: A perspective. In: U. Drill and P. Lazar (eds) *Cutaneous Toxicity.* Academic Press, New York.

317. Weisberger, A.S. 1958. Tumor inhibition by a sulfhydryl blocking agent related to an active principle of garlic. *Cancer Research* Dec. 18:1301-8.

318. Weiss, S.J., Lampert, M.B., Test, S.T. 1983. Long-lived oxidants generated by human neutrophils. *Science* 222:626.

319. Werbach, M.R. 1987. *Nutritional Influences on Illness.* Third Line Press Inc., Tarzana, CA.

320. Westrick, E. Shapiro, A., et al. 1988. Dietary tryptophan reverses alcohol-induced impairment of facial recognition but not verbal recall. *Alc. Clin. Exp.* 12:531-33.

321. Whitacre, M.E., Combs, G.F. 1983. Selenium and mitochondrial integrity in the pancreas of the chick. *J. Nutr.* 113:1972.

322. White, J.W., Jr. 1976. Relative significance of dietary source of nitrate and nitrite. *J. Agri. Food. Chem.* 23:886-891.

323. White, J.W., Jr. 1976. Correlation relative significance of dietary source of nitrate and nitrite. *J. Agri. Food. Chem.* 24:202.

324. Wilkins, J.R.III, Reiches, N.A., Kruse, C.W. 1979. Organic chemical contaminants in drinking water and cancer. *Am. J. Epidemiol.* 110:420-448.

325. Willett, W., et al. 1976. Selenium and human health. *Nutr. Rev.* 34(11):347.

326. Williams, S.R. 1973. *Review of Nutrition and Diet Therapy.* C.V. Mosby Co., St. Louis.

327. Williams, R.J. 1971. *Nutrition Against Disease.* Pitman, New York.

328. Williams, R.J. 1980. *Alcoholism — The Nutritional Approach.* Univ. Texas Press, Austin.

329. Wimhurst, J.M., Manchester, K.L. 1972. Comparison of ability of Mg and Mn to activate the key enzymes of glycolysis. *F.E.R.S. Letters* 27:321-6.

330. Winitz, M., et al. 1964. Effect of dietary carbohydrate on serum cholesterol levels. *Archives of Biochemistry and Biophysics* 108:576-79.

331. Wissler, R.W. 1976. Current status of regression studies. *Athero. Rev.* 3:213.

332. Wissler, R.W. 1979. Evidence for regression of advanced atherosclerotic plaques. *Arteriosclerosis* 5:398.

333. Wolf, G. 1982. Is dietary carotene an anti-cancer agent? *Nutr. Rev.* 40:257.

334. Wright, A., et al. 1986. Food allergy or intolerance in severe recurrent aphthous ulceration of the mouth. *Br. Med. J.* 292(6530):1237-8.

335. Wurtman, J.J., Zeisel, S.H. 1982. Carbohydrate craving in obese people. *Inter. J. Eat. Dis.* 1:4.

336. Wurtman, R.J., Wurtman, J.J. 1983. Physiological and Behavioral Effects of Food Constituents. *Nutrition and the Brain.* Vol. 6. Raven Press, N.Y.

337. Wynder, E. 1987. Amount and type of fat/fiber in nutritional carcinogenesis. *Prev. Med. 16:451-459.*

338. Yanick, P., Jaffe, R. 1988. *Clinical Chemistry and Nutrition Guidebook: a Physician's Desk Reference.* Vol. 1 T&H Publishing.

339. Yudkin, J., Edelman, I., Hough, L. (eds.) 1971. *Sugar: Chemical, Biological, and Nutritional Aspects of Sucrose.* Daniel Davey, Hartford, Conn.

340. Yudkin, J. 1957. Diet and coronary thrombosis. Hypothesis and fact. *Lancet* 11:155-62.

341. Yudkin, J., et al. 1986. Dietary sucrose affects plasma HDL cholesterol concentrations in young men. *Ann. Nutr. Metab.* 30(4):261-66.

342. Ziegler, R., et al. 1984. Dietary carotene, vitamin A and risk of lung cancer among white men in New Jersey. *J. Nat'l. Can. Inst.* 73:1429.

343. Zimmerman, B. 1979. Do onions and garlic prevent thrombi? *Mod. Med.* 23.

344. Zioudrou, C., Klee, W.A. 1979. Possible roles of peptides derived from food proteins in brain function. *Nutrition in the Brain* 4:125-52.

345. Zulik, R., et al. 1972. Death cap poisoning. *Lancet* 2:288.

Index

Vitamin E and, 104
water quality and, 96
Candida Albicans, 36, 234-235. See also
Yeast infections
Caper-Almond Salad, 196
Carrot and Avocado Dressing, 215
Carrot and Cream Cooler, 213
Carrots Piquant, 194
Cardiac arrhythmia. See Heart disease
Carlson Laboratories, 129
Carnitine. See Amino Acids
Catalase, 52
Cells
atrophy of, 41
damage to, 95-96
epithelial, 23
hydrogenated fats and, 35
membranes of, 25, 42
mitochondria, 143
Cheese, 151
Chemicals. See Additives
Chicken. See Poultry
Chicken "Cure a Cold" Soup, 189-190
Chlorella, 86, 129, 223,230. See also Beta
carotene
alcoholism and, 138, 139
definition of, 110
liver protection and, 91
Wakasa, 240
Chlorella Cooler, 212, 213
Chloroflurocarbons
ozone and, 51
Chlorophyll, 110
Cholesterol, 87, 252-253
alcohol consumption and, 80
diet and, 65-66
discussion of blood levels, 247-249
HDL, 68, 70
healthy fats and, 141-142
heart disease and, 63
hypothyroidism and, 23
LDL, 68
levels of, 64-65
sources of, 65
Choline, 93-94
Chlorophyll, 110
Chromium, 11, 233
blood sugar and, 23
heart disease and, 82
Chromium picolinate, 82
Cigarette smoking, 39, 80, 235
Circulatory system, 26
Coenzyme Q-10 25, 80, 88
Cold Sores, 222-223
Colds, 222
Colon

cancer, 84
toxic, 40
Constipation, 87, 90, 223
Copper, 233
Crab Cakes, 180
Crackerless Meat Loaf, 168
Cranberry Juice Creamy Surprise, 211-212
Creamy Garlic-Avocado Dressing, 219
Creatinine
discussion of blood levels, 242-243

D

Depression. See Psychological Disorders
Diarrhea
remedies for, 224
Diced Fruit in a Bowl, 209
Diabetes, 16, 87, 107
foods and herbs for, 236
hydrogenated fats and, 36
nutrients for, 235-236
sugar and, 117
Diet. See also Food; Nutritional
deficiencies
common deficiencies, 10
effects of poor, 3-4
low-fiber, 87
Standard American, 10-11
Digestive system. See also Constipation;
Diarrhea
disturbances in, 23
diverticulitis, 87
enzymes, 118
essential fatty acids and, 22
foods for, 87
health of, 22
hypothyroidism and, 23
stress and, 85-86
vegetables and, 109
Dilled Broccoli/Cauliflower Combo, 205
Dips
recipes for, 216-219
Diseases. See individual entries
Diuretics, 13, 74
Drinks
recipes for, 210-215
Drugs, non-prescription, 12
antihistamines, 13
aspirin, 6,
laxatives, 13, 164
Drugs, prescription, 5. See also Diuretics;
Birth Control Pills, 13
nutritional deficiencies and, 11-14
premature death and, 16
toxicity of, 16

heart disease and, 82
psychological disorders and, 120

W — Z

Walnut/Pine Nut Stuffed Onions, 200
Water, 96-101. *See also* Water purifiers
Watercress Salad, 191-192
Watercress-Tomato Soup, 188
Water pills. *See* Diuretics
Water purifiers, 98-100
Waterfier, 99-101
Wheat. See Grains
White Fish in Lemon-Dill Sauce, 175

Yeast, 24, 40, 41
Yeast infection, 23, 119. See also Candida
  Albicans
Yogurt
  recipes for, 221-222
Yogurt-Cucumber Salad, 196
Yohimbe Root. See Herbs
YSK International, 240

Zinc, 11, 14, 230, 233
  alcoholism and, 139
  bran and, 255
  cell repair and, 23
  deficiency of, 22, 139
  impotence and, 227
  prostate and, 227
  skin and, 19, 228
Zucchini Canoes, 204-205
Zucchini in Olive Oil, 203

ABOUT DR. IGRAM

Dr. Cass Igram is a physician, healer, and expert in nutritional therapy. He received his B.S. degree at the University of Northern Iowa in biology and chemistry. He received his degree at the University of Osteopathic Medicine and Health Sciences, Des Moines, Iowa. Dr. Igram is a respected lecturer and educator. He specializes in teaching both doctors and the public about nutritional treatments.

His accomplishments include having his own radio show in the Chicago metropolitan area, conducting educational seminars for doctors, chiropractors, and healing specialists of all types, and designing methods for the drug-free treatment of disease.

Dr. Igram formerly owned and operated the Igram Preventive Medical Center where he successfully treated hundreds of patients with illnesses ranging from heart disease to psychosis without using drugs.

ABOUT JUDY K. GRAY

Judy K. Gray received her Masters of Science degree in Nutrition from Central Missouri State University. She has been active in the field of nutrition for the past 19 years as an independent practitioner, in medical clinics, and in private hospitals. Ms. Gray has appeared on many television and radio shows which included "Nutrition Hotline" with Doctor Igram. She has lived abroad and has travelled extensively throughout the world observing and learning about human nutrition.

Ms. Gray was formerly Director of Nutrition in a Chicago area hospital. She has lectured, conducted seminars, facilitated corporate wellness programs, and written extensively on health and nutrition topics. Ms. Gray is President of the American Institute of Curative Medicine and consultant for Nutrition Testing and Consulting Services.

Notes

Notes